AF840575

Coding and Documentation Compliance for the ICD and DSM

Coding and Documentation Compliance for the ICD and DSM provides professionals, professors, and students with a logical and practical way of understanding a difficult topic in healthcare for the clinician: coding. Established professionals will find the tools they need to comply with the ICD series, HIPAA, and integrated care models. Professors and students will appreciate having a systemized, standardized approach to teaching and learning the more complex aspects of ICD compliance. The interplay between the ICD and DSM manuals is also explicated in clear terms.

Lisette Wright, MA, is a licensed psychologist, EHR systems administrator, and recipient of certificates in health information systems and corporate compliance. Her curriculum has been taught to more than 13,000 clinicians nationally since 2013.

S. M. Tobias, MFA, MSW, has a background in writing and mental health and has been in the healthcare field for over twenty years. She currently owns and operates a group private practice in Minnesota.

Angela Hickman, CPC, CPMA, CPCO, CEDC, is an AHIMA-approved ICD-10-CM/PCS trainer and a senior management consultant. She has more than twenty years of experience in healthcare, from training medical providers to revenue cycle optimization and coding compliance.

Coding and Documentation Compliance for the ICD and DSM

A Comprehensive Guide for Clinicians

LISETTE WRIGHT, S. M. TOBIAS, AND
ANGELA HICKMAN

Routledge
Taylor & Francis Group
NEW YORK AND LONDON

First published 2017
by Routledge
711 Third Avenue, New York, NY 10017

and by Routledge
2 Park Square, Milton Park, Abingdon, Oxon, OX14 4RN

Routledge is an imprint of the Taylor & Francis Group, an informa business

© 2017 Lisette Wright, S. M. Tobias, and Angela Hickman

The right of Lisette Wright, S. M. Tobias, and Angela Hickman to be identified as authors of this work has been asserted by them in accordance with sections 77 and 78 of the Copyright, Designs and Patents Act 1988.

All rights reserved. The purchase of this copyright material confers the right on the purchasing institution to photocopy or download pages which bear the eResources icon and a copyright line at the bottom of the page. No other parts of this book may be reprinted or reproduced or utilised in any form or by any electronic, mechanical, or other means, now known or hereafter invented, including photocopying and recording, or in any information storage or retrieval system, without permission in writing from the publishers.

Trademark notice: Product or corporate names may be trademarks or registered trademarks, and are used only for identification and explanation without intent to infringe.

Library of Congress Cataloging in Publication Data
A catalog record for this book has been requested.

ISBN: 978-1-138-67765-4 (hbk)
ISBN: 978-1-138-67766-1 (pbk)
ISBN: 978-1-315-56357-2 (ebk)

Typeset in Dante and Avenir
by Keystroke, Neville Lodge, Tettenhall, Wolverhampton

Contents

Author Biography

Lisette Wright, MA, Licensed Psychologist. Lisette's background includes working for mental health agencies, as an independent consultant for behavioral health organizations, and as the administrator of a behavioral health clinic. She is currently an EHR systems administrator, provider, national consultant, and educator. Since obtaining a Certificate in Clinical Information Systems, Lisette has specialized in the Health Information Technology sector of behavioral health. Her focus has been helping organizations prepare, choose, and implement HIT and Health Care Reform initiatives into their practices. She has trained more than 13,000 clinicians across the United States on this curriculum. Lisette recently obtained her Certificate in Corporate Compliance from the Charlotte School of Law.

Lisette's interests include humanitarian work in Africa. She is active in the non-profit organization The Kisangaji Project, which she founded in 2008 after visiting the remote village in Tanzania, East Africa. Owner and Executive Director of Behavioral Health Solutions, she can be reached via www.behavioralhealthsolutionsmn.com

Preface

This book is disciplinary agnostic, which means it can be utilized by graduate programs and healthcare operations involving: psychology, counseling, social work, alcohol and drug programs, psychiatric education, healthcare administration modules, and more. Existing and newly minted behavioral health clinicians, administrators, compliance officials, auditors, and others will appreciate the clear, practical, and straightforward presentation of the information in this textbook.

The book is written mainly for graduate-level students in the behavioral sciences. However, anyone interested in the standardization of healthcare and the provision of quality behavioral health service delivery—including administrators, policy-makers, and third party entities such as healthcare payers—will deem this book essential.

In the course of the book, the following two sets of terms are used interchangeably or in certain given contexts: practitioner, clinician, or provider; and client, consumer, or patient. Read these within the context of your own understanding and language. While the medical industry historically has utilized a defined process for coding and documentation, the behavioral healthcare industry has not. Therefore, it is recognized by the authors of this book that by asking behavioral health clinicians to use the ICD-10-CM Tabular List of Diseases and Injuries (i.e. the Tabular Index), much less an Alphabetic Index first, requires a seismic paradigm shift in the industry.

It is highly recommended to the behavioral health industry that clinicians must verify their assigned diagnosis codes in the Tabular Index *and* follow the ICD-10-CM Coding and Documentation Guidelines. Doing so will bring the behavioral healthcare field closer to being compliant, adherent, and ultimately, contributing more precisely to population health.

While the ICD-10 is an international diagnostic coding system, the authors live in the USA. Therefore, unless we are referring to the ICD series, or ICD-10 specifically in the global context, we will refer to the ICD-10-CM throughout the book. Every attempt is made to give consideration to the context in which "ICD-10" is used, and therefore the reader may wonder why they sometimes see "ICD-10" and "ICD-10-CM."

Because coding processes vary across organization, regions, providers, and settings, a disclaimer is needed: the "correct" coding process is subject to the procedures of your workplace and the specific nature of your work. Workplaces need to have policies and procedures in place to help clinicians with the more subjective aspects of coding and documentation. Finally, the diagnosis assignment of clients is the responsibility of the clinician.

Abbreviations and Entities Referred to in this Text

The following terms and abbreviations are used throughout the text. Their descriptions are very brief and are not all-encompassing. Please feel free to research the items further.

AHIMA (American Health Information Management Association). Large trade association in the USA of health information practice professionals who provide research, tools, and resources to the industry.

AHRQ (Agency for Healthcare Research and Quality). A division of the US Department of Health and Human Services that focuses on providing the healthcare industry with evidence-based best practice research and recommendations.

APA (American Psychiatric Association). A US-based trade association for psychiatrists. APA has a publishing division, of which the DSM series has been one of their leading best sellers.

CDC (Centers for Disease Control and Prevention). The CDC is a component of the Department of Health and Human Services. CDC increases the health security of our nation and is the nation's health protection agency.

CDI (Clinical Documentation Improvement). A process of reviewing medical records for purposes of improving the clinical quality, content, and integrity of the record. This process can be iterative ("Continual CDI") and can be performed by any number of entities, both within and outside the organization.

CMS (Centers for Medicare & Medicaid Services). The Centers for Medicare & Medicaid Services is a federal agency within the United States Department of Health and Human Services that administers the Medicare program and works in partnership with state governments to administer Medicaid, the State Children's Health Insurance Program, and health insurance portability standards. In addition to these programs, CMS has other responsibilities, including the administrative simplification standards from the Health Insurance Portability and Accountability Act of 1996.

CP (Compliance Program). A formal ethics and compliance program within healthcare organizations, required by the Affordable Care Act. This program has a formal structure, set of responsibilities for oversight, training and education, and monitoring and auditing of the organization's workforce.

CPC (Certified Professional Coder). A designated, certified individual in professional coding for the purposes of coding and documentation compliance in the healthcare industry. These individuals are trained and certified in all healthcare coding sets, evaluation and management principles, and in documentation. Largely employed by the medical industry, behavioral health organizations are recognizing the need to employ CPCs.

DSM (Diagnostic and Statistical Manual of Mental Disorders). The DSM is published by the American Psychiatric Association (APA) and offers a common language and standard criteria for the classification of mental disorders. The DSM is now in its fifth edition, with DSM-5 published in May 2013.

EHR (Electronic Health Record). An electronic health record is an official health record for an individual that can be shared among multiple facilities and agencies. An EHR is a digital version of a medical record. You may also hear the term "EMR" which stands for electronic medical record.

EMR (Electronic Medical Record). EMR is a generic term long used by providers to refer to a computerized patient record. Discrete EMR systems are used to improve practices, basically replacing paper charts with computerized records. They are different from EHRs in that they do not have the capability to exchange information electronically with other systems.

HIM (Health Information Management). The acquisition, management, and protection of health information in any form, electronic or paper records.

HIT (Health Information Technology). HIT is the utilization of information technology (computer sciences) in the health care industry. Before the introduction of HIT, most medical records and related ancillary information were kept on paper. HIT enables the sharing of information between computer systems, leading to increased efficiency of workflows and safety for clients.

ICD (**The International Classification of Diseases**). ICD is the international standard diagnostic tool for epidemiology, health management, and clinical purposes. It is used to monitor the incidence and prevalence of diseases and other health problems, providing a picture of the general health situation of countries and populations. In addition to enabling the storage and retrieval of diagnostic information for clinical, epidemiological, and quality purposes, these records also provide the basis for the compilation of national mortality and morbidity statistics by WHO member states. Finally, ICD is used for reimbursement and resource allocation decision-making by countries. ICD is currently under revision, through an ongoing revision process, and the anticipated release date for ICD-11 is 2018 (at the time of this writing), although many experts believe the release will be much later.

ICD-10 CDDG (**ICD's Clinical Descriptions and Diagnostic Guidelines**). This is a book published by the WHO and it contains the clinical criteria for clinicians to reference when assigning ICD-10 diagnoses. Also known as the Blue Book, it was publishing in 1992 and is currently undergoing revision to align with the upcoming ICD-11.

IHTSDO (**International Health Terminology Standards Development**). Based in Denmark, this international organization is comprised of members who are committed to standardizing health terminology across the globe. They own, administer, and develop the Systematized Nomenclature of Medicine, Clinical Terms, or SNOMED CT.

NCHS (**National Center for Health Statistics**). As the nation's principal health statistics agency, the NCHS compiles statistical information to guide actions and policies to improve the health of all people. NCHS is a unique public resource for health information—a critical element of public health and health policy. Health statistics allow us to: follow the health status of a population, track healthcare delivery trends and health disparities, identify health problems, evaluate the impact of health policy, and support biomedical research, to name a few.

NLM (**National Library of Medicine**). The NLM, a branch of the US National Institute of Health, operates the **UMLS** (**Unified Medical Language System**). The UMLS integrates and distributes key terminology, classification and coding standards in the healthcare system. This includes SNOMED CT.

OIG (**Office of the Inspector General**). The OIG is the office charged with integrity investigations that is part of the US Federal Department of Health and Human Services. Its mission is to fight fraud, waste, and abuse, and to protect the beneficiaries of programs under its purview.

SNOMED CT (Systematized Nomenclature of Medicine, Clinical Terms). Owned and distributed by IHTSDO, SNOMED CT is the most comprehensive and precise system of healthcare clinical terminology (including for the veterinary sciences) in the world.

WHO (World Health Organization). The World Health Organization is headquartered in Geneva, Switzerland, and focuses on international public health. Priorities and tasks of the WHO include: moving health systems towards universal health coverage, policy, research, and academics.

Acknowledgments

Beth Tschopp: Researcher, Reviewer, and Colleague
Caitlin Cocker: Researcher
Val Roster Martin: Researcher
Laura Morgan: Researcher, Curriculum Content Improvements
Virna Little: Endorsement and Reviewer
Mike Lardieri: Endorsement and Reviewer
Dr. Varun Choudhary: Endorsement and Reviewer
Christine Polson: Certified Professional Coder, SME
Kasey Giordano: SME
Dr. Michael Sterns: SME
Serafina Versaggi: SNOMED CT SME
Rennie Joshi: Researcher and Reviewer
College Hospitals, Costa Mesa and Cerritos, California

For my parents (LW)

Introduction

This book aims to change the way behavioral health clinicians think about and assign mental health diagnoses to their clients. While seemingly a banal topic, the International Classification of Diseases (ICD) coding and documentation system is actually quite multi-faceted, informative and useful in our day-to-day work with clients and within integrated healthcare models. Embedded into our health information technology solutions, the ICD series gives us a powerful resource that has the potential to change behavioral health service delivery as we know it.

Since the inception of the ICD-10-CM, and for the first time in US history, clinicians in the behavioral healthcare system now have a critical tool to electronically track, mitigate, and possibly prevent suicide. Additionally, we now have a way to comprehensively look at a client's entire health status with a one-page snapshot: a comprehensive summary that informs us of all the medical conditions our clients experience that perpetuate, contribute to, or complicate their mental health situation. We now have access to a common language and terminology that links clients' mental health care to their medical care. The integration of a uniform coding and documentation system underscores the imperative that behavioral health cannot be separated from medical health. It is now our job to embrace and adopt this holistic approach into our culture in behavioral health. The availability of the entire diagnostic code set contained in the ICD series can help us improve population health, reduce the number of suicides, and improve the overall quality of care we provide to clients. To do this effectively, we need to be vigilant that *all* ICD-10-CM codes are available to us in the Electronic Health Record diagnosis section.

The Diagnostic and Statistical Manual (DSM) has historically been the predominant clinical manual utilized in the behavioral health industry for diagnosing and treating clients in the USA; it has additionally been the system exclusively taught to graduate students and burgeoning clinicians in the American mental health field. A review of the available textbooks for graduate-level study of diagnostic criteria supports the ubiquity of DSM curriculum in the field. The workforce in the USA must now utilize the ICD series, and it has become imperative to have a *standardized ICD curriculum* and teaching materials available to our graduate programs nationwide. One hope for this book is that it becomes the standard teaching tool for newly-emerging clinicians in behavioral health worldwide. Shaping knowledge and excellent clinical documentation, habits, and coding practices is imperative to workforce readiness. However, the majority of practitioners and administrators do not understand the complexity of the ICD system, in that it contains diagnostic, coding, and documentation guidelines that behavioral health clinicians are now mandated to use. The ICD is not just about assigning the "correct diagnosis." It is a comprehensive, research-based, worldwide system for all healthcare providers.

Clinicians in the USA have historically relied upon the DSM series for diagnosing and conceptualizing the mental health of their clients. However, the DSM series is limited, designed by a select group, not open source or free, and not comprehensive with regards to assigning diagnoses for all conditions that affect our clients, including medical conditions and psychosocial stressors. The DSM series, while utilized in some but not all countries, is not the global standard for mental health diagnoses. In fact, having two classification systems, with different diagnostic criteria, that do not align and create confusion is arguably counter-productive and certainly not efficient. The authors recognize that not everyone will agree with this premise and that the allegiance to the DSM series evokes strong reactions in the industry.

Despite the divisiveness, all healthcare entities covered by the Health Insurance Portability and Accountability Act (HIPAA) in the USA are now mandated to use the ICD series, and the DSM is not considered "HIPAA compliant." In fact, some would argue that the DSM is not a coding system at all; it is a diagnostic guide to assigning mental health and substance use conditions to those who receive healthcare services. The problem is that so many clinicians in America "believe" that the DSM is a code set, and is the "only" option for diagnosing clients. This is not true, and the ICD series now gives us a standardized, comprehensive, integrated model and corresponding diagnostic guidelines for assigning applicable diagnoses to our clients. This will be far more important for health information technology systems and Continuity of

Care Documents (CCDs) where the text or narrative portion of the medical record is not reviewed or shared. Why is this so important and why should we care?

Healthcare worldwide is fast marching towards standardized, interoperable, interchangeable, and easily accessible information about diseases and conditions for purposes of research, population health, and the delivery of healthcare services. The ICD series is, and has been, used internationally. Having one classification system and one set of diagnostic criteria across all healthcare disciplines is critical for achieving global health initiatives. It is anticipated that with the new comprehensive care delivery model of Certified Community Behavioral Health Centers (CCBHCs) in the USA, the associated requirements will only be met by the full utilization and acceptance of the ICD series. The CCBHC model will be the new gold standard for care in the behavioral health industry, regardless of practice setting.

This book is written not just for the practicing behavioral health clinician; it is written for the entire behavioral health industry: community mental health centers, academia, administrators, policy-makers, solo-practitioners, as well as third parties such as regulators, payers, and accrediting bodies. This book is based on several premises and a few recommendations for the behavioral healthcare industry, which are relevant both for clinical practice and for administrative purposes.

Some of the premises of this book include:

- Behavioral health providers, in order to be treated as equal compatriots in the healthcare industry who are bound by HIPAA, must begin to code and document like the rest of the healthcare industry.
- The DSM series is simply one option for obtaining diagnostic guidelines to arrive at a behavioral health diagnosis. It is not a code book. The ICD series also contains diagnostic guidelines for arriving at behavioral health diagnoses and codes. The diagnosis guidelines for the ICD series align with the ICD diagnoses and clinicians may find utilizing one set of materials less confusing that using two disparate manuals.
- Behavioral health clinicians must learn how to speak the same language as other healthcare disciplines. While some have argued that this translates into "the medicalization of mental health," others have proposed that this standardization will validate our status as key providers in consumer care.
- We can only provide quality healthcare service delivery and achieve stellar epidemiology and research results when we use common, standardized, language and code sets that relate to each other in a way that holds the same meaning for everyone.

- To meet objectives of integrated healthcare, behavioral health clinicians will need to figure out how to code for medical and self-harm diagnoses to leverage health information technologies. We have a tool to prevent suicides (i.e. the X-codes), and to not use these codes is a disservice to all those who struggle with hopelessness. We used to notate medical conditions on Axis III in the DSM-IV-TR. Now that the multi-axial system is gone, how can we comfortably code for medical diagnoses when we are not medical doctors yet are held responsible for integrated, value-based care? Clinicians will need policies and procedures in place to help guide them when assigning medical diagnoses to their clients.
- Changing an entire culture and inter-generational approach to conceptualizing and formulating psychiatric cases for treatment purposes will take time and dedication. It is the authors' belief that this integration must start in our graduate schools, which are training the upcoming behavioral healthcare workforce. We hope this book is the beginning of this change.

There are a few further important points to make:

- Behavioral health is just like any other medical specialty, except that the outcomes of intervention are much more difficult to quantify. Any movement in this direction is an improvement, and utilization of the ICD series will help tremendously with this objective.
- That said, it is unlikely that behavioral health will "think" and use the ICD coding system in the same way the medical industry does (e.g. through the utilization of certified professional coders to assign the diagnosis code). To that end, we are recommending that behavioral health moves closer to integration by following as many of the procedures utilized in the medical industry as possible.
- The ICD series, in particular the ICD-10, is not new. In fact, it has been in existence since the 1990s. Soon, we will have ICD-11, ICD-11-CM and the new ICD-11 Clinical Descriptions and Diagnostic Guidelines (CDDG). This is a very exciting time in the history of behavioral health as we will, for the first time in history, have a truly compatible, updated, and congruent set of reference materials that are open source and free to use when working with clients. There will be no more discrepancies to contend with and hopefully the confusion for all stakeholders will dissipate with the embracing of the entire ICD series.
- A draft version of the new ICD-11 CDDG is available and open to the entire community of interested stakeholders. This manual, reflective of an international, transparent contribution process by all, will be the most

current itemization of symptoms and clinical descriptions to support ICD-11 mental and behavioral health diagnoses.
- Systematized Nomenclature of Medicine, Clinical Terms (SNOMED CT) is already in use across the globe. While not a large part of this book, SNOMED CT is discussed at a basic level to help all behavioral health clinicians understand the implications of it in their daily practices.

Finally, this curriculum was written by individuals who have worked in the behavioral health and medical industry their entire careers. We are subject-matter experts and have clinical backgrounds. The curriculum and book are written in such a way that this difficult material should be comprehensible to most everyone. From the new graduate student, the seasoned clinician, to the clinic chief operating officer or administrator, this book provides a massive amount of information presented in an understandable way that makes sense to those in the behavioral health industry.

The chapters are written to be cumulative and they build on the information presented in a very specific order. There is a method to the curriculum and while the initial two chapters may seem "optional," they indeed are not. In order to understand how computer systems, electronic health records (EHRs), diagnosing and billing actually work, one must understand the context for the challenges that face those in the US behavioral healthcare industry.

Chapters 1 and 2 provide the reader with an introduction to the ICD series. They will also begin to help the reader understand where the "coding and documentation" guidelines come from and delineate the purpose they serve in healthcare. Understanding how they work will also be imperative for those who need to make decisions about policies and procedures for their organization. Essentially, we will need to take as much standardized information and guidelines as possible and adapt them in a way that maintains fidelity to the intent of the guidelines for coding and documentation.

The middle part of the book details what we need to know about the ICD codes and how to use them. Chapters 3 and 4 will go into detail about the diagnosis codes, where they originate, and their utilization. We also specifically talk about the clinical diagnostic criteria differences between the DSM series and the ICD series and how having two disparate systems can be problematic and confusing. Certainly, there is a call to have one standard coding and documentation system across all healthcare specialties leading to value-based, integrated service delivery. You will see why the ICD series is best equipped to meet this objective when we discuss medical and suicidal codes in the book.

A chapter on SNOMED CT is included in this book because we will be hearing more and more about SNOMED CT moving into the future. SNOMED CT is a complex topic, and every attempt was made to have the chapter address these basic questions: what is SNOMED CT and how will it apply to the future of behavioral health practice? The chapter serves as an overview and introduction only.

We close the book with a section on compliance, including thoughts and recommendations about policies and procedures to help standardize and improve the quality of behavioral healthcare delivery. This book will challenge the status quo by suggesting that we transition to a unified system, with corresponding clinical diagnostic guidelines, which ultimately brings us into alignment with the rest of the healthcare industry.

We hope that by the end of the book, you will be as passionate about this subject as we are.

Laying the Groundwork 1

In our current, American healthcare climate, it is imperative for behavioral health providers to collaborate with other specialty medical professionals, such as nurses and physicians. Clinically integrated service delivery and value-based care are now essential in the behavioral health service delivery industry. Some critics have referred to this development as the "medicalization of mental health." With recent changes, including the newly-mandated adherence to coding and documentation guidelines, behavioral healthcare clinicians must now work more in tandem with their medical counterparts to improve their systemic and practical approaches to these topics. Educating newly emerging clinicians as they enter the field is the next, important step in ensuring a current and next generation of clinical competence.

We are at a monumental crossroads in the USA in regard to behavioral health diagnostic classification systems. For most licensed clinicians who have practiced prior to 2013, they are familiar with the DSM-IV-TR codes. In 2015–16, students were beginning to graduate from our schools educated only with the knowledge of the DSM-5 manual and codes. Some, but relatively few, were taught about the DSM-IV-TR and ICD-9 series. Due to this discrepancy in curriculums, we have a workforce of behavioral health clinicians who have learned and practiced with a multitude of differing code sets, diagnostic criteria, manuals, and expectations. This lack of coherence has relegated the education and training of newer clinicians to already-stretched workplace systems and employers. Until now, there has been an absence of a comprehensive, standardized textbook that has been distributed to explain this complex situation.

Behavioral health practitioners have historically been behind the times in regard to the Health Insurance Portability and Accountability Act (HIPAA), passed by Congress in 1996. As HIPAA-covered entities, behavioral health clinicians are required to adhere to the ICD-10-CM Official Guidelines for Coding and Reporting put forth by the Centers for Medicare & Medicaid Services (CMS). These documents are updated at least annually. Yet, coding and documentation guidelines have historically not been expected of, or enforced in, behavioral health settings, clinics, or even taught in graduate schools. In fact, many behavioral healthcare clinicians are not aware that guidelines for coding and documentation exist. Accreditation bodies, auditors, and other regulatory agencies are now looking at the provision of behavioral health services with new eyes, ones that indicate we need to prioritize our standards and improve practices.

Coding and documentation compliance also relates to revenue cycle processes and includes discussions about CPT codes (i.e. Current Procedural Terminology, the code set published by the Amercian Medical Association), documentation requirements, medical necessity, coding manuals, and compliance with CMS procedures for billing behavioral health services properly. While intrinsically related, these items are not directly discussed in this book. However, it is important to keep in mind the following items:

- "Improper payments," as defined by CMS and the US Department of Health and Human Service Program Integrity Plan, include payments made for services not supported by the documentation.
- CPT codes explicitly define what constitutes a "service."
- CMS's annual Payment Error Rate Measurement (PERM) reports frequently find that a significant portion of improper Medicaid payments result from documentation errors, insufficient documentation, and policy violations such as not documenting start and stop times.
- Regulators and auditors look at all aspects of documentation and coding, not just as it relates to the ICD and DSM.
- This book focuses on coding and documentation compliance processes as they relate to the ICD and DSM, not the rest of the revenue cycle per se.

Integrated care models and the government's recent emphasis on legitimizing behavioral health concerns to the level of physical health have placed a heightened expectation on the behavioral health industry to improve their coding and documentation. CMS, coupled with the World Health Organization's International Classification of Diseases (ICD) system, provides the behavioral health system with all the necessary tools to become compatriots with the medical industry in the healthcare delivery system. Understanding the ICD-10-CM and its relationship to the DSM is critical to all stakeholders in the behavioral health industry, including clinicians, administrators, students, and third parties who possess fiscal interest in the behavioral healthcare field.

Understanding the International Classification of Diseases

What is the ICD-10-CM and its Use in the USA

Historically, behavioral healthcare clinicians have typically utilized a diagnostic manual called the *Diagnostic and Statistical Manual of Mental Disorders* (DSM, currently in its fifth edition), published by the American Psychiatric Association. Alongside the DSM, providers in the medical field have also utilized another classification system, the ICD, published by the World Health Organization (WHO). Each classification system has its own, unique set of diagnostic clinical criteria necessary to assign a certain diagnostic condition to a client; both systems contain essential information pertinent for insurance reimbursement, coding, documentation, compliance, and research. These specific systems both include the actual diagnostic codes for several purposes: claims, documentation, and research. Yet these two systems do not currently align, which creates confusion for clinicians, billers, and payers alike.

The ICD is an international tool and standard for defining and reporting diseases and health conditions. As stated by the WHO (2016):

> The ICD is the standard diagnostic tool for epidemiology, health management and clinical purposes. This includes the analysis of the general health situation of population groups. It is used to monitor the incidence and prevalence of diseases and other health problems.

The WHO establishes which ICD series, or volume, is current. The forty-third World Health Assembly approved the tenth version (ICD-10) for use in 1990. All member organizations of the WHO use the ICD series for their healthcare needs, and yet each member state can adapt and adopt the ICD to its own needs and timing. Most member nations of the WHO, consisting of 117 countries, adopted the ICD-10 for use early on in the 1990s. It was not until much later, in October 2015, that the USA officially adopted the ICD-10-CM for use.

The ICD-10 is currently undergoing a revision process by the WHO, and it is hoped that the World Health Assembly will approve the next version—the ICD-11—in 2018. While the WHO may formally approve a new version of the ICD, the actual timing for adoption can vary across member states. It is also thought that the release of ICD-11 will not actually happen in 2018 and that it could take an additional number of years before its release. The USA was one of the last member nations to formally implement the ICD-10, some 25 years after the World Health Assembly approved it. The process for implementation in the USA is especially complicated, thus creating some of the delay in implementing the current code set in a timely manner. We may not see the adoption of ICD-11-CM in the USA for more than a decade from this writing, leaving clinicians with confounding diagnostic systems until then.

Each member state is permitted to adopt the ICD to meet the needs of its own country. In addition, each member state can establish its own "version" of the ICD to distinguish it from the WHO's adopted version of the ICD. In the USA, the ICD is distinguished by using the initials "CM" after the current version number. CM stands for "Clinical Modification," and it is formally referenced as the ICD-10-CM, which indicates that the codes are US specific. Other countries have different versions of the ICD-10, which reflect each country's specific cultural norms and/or adjustment to certain diagnostic language.

An example of how the USA has modified the ICD-10-CM language for its own use is reflected in Table 1.1. The term "mental retardation" was struck from the ICD-10 and replaced with the term "intellectual disability" in the US version ICD-10-CM when President Obama signed the Rosa Act in 2010. Table 1.1 reflects the language differences:

Table 1.1 Language Differences Between the ICD and DSM

WHO ICD-10, Chapter 5 Clinical Descriptions	The US ICD-10-CM, Tabular Index Listing
F70-79: "Mental Retardation"	F70-F79: "Intellectual Disability"

Two US entities, the Centers for Disease Control and Prevention (CDC) and the National Center for Health Statistics (NCHS), largely oversee the maintenance and development of the official ICD-10-CM in the USA, with oversight by the US Department of Health and Human Services. It is updated twice a year, based on processes for proposing and vetting changes to the ICD. The most recent itemization of the ICD can be found on the CDC website: www.cdc.gov/nchs/icd/icd10cm.htm#icd2016.

A formal process for reviewing the WHO's ICD and adapting it to conform to our own cultural norms exists in the USA. CMS, along with the CDC, has established a Coordination and Maintenance Committee to oversee the process of adapting the ICD for use in the USA. Most recently, this committee was called the "ICD-10 Coordination and Maintenance Committee." This committee provides a public forum to discuss proposed changes to the WHO's ICD for utilization specific to the USA's needs. Public committee meetings are venues for input and recommendations. During these meetings, individuals or representative stakeholder groups are allocated times to discuss proposed changes to the official ICD. Occasionally, a person or group may present a short proposal for a certain diagnosis that is not currently recognized. A recent example of this was the proposal by a stakeholder group to include the diagnosis "Hoarding Disorder" in the official ICD-10-CM listing as it was not originally in the ICD-10-CM for the first two years after ICD-10-CM went live.

Final decisions regarding acceptance, rejection, or changes to either procedural or diagnostic categories in the ICD are the responsibility of the US Department of Health and Human Services, with the final decision rendered upon further review. It is critical to understand this process for a variety of reasons, including:

- The current ICD may differ from the current US version.
- Adding "CM" to the title identifies the US version.
- Despite concerted efforts to collect global health statistics for public health and incidence reporting, some discrepancies between countries may be found due to regional differences.
- The USA approaches changes to the WHO's ICD seriously and only adopts changes after considerable input from subject matter experts and stakeholders.

Despite some of the differences in the ICD variations across member nations, the structure and content of codes, diagnoses, and classifications remain consistent. This consistency enables WHO member nations to collect and analyze data globally, thus leading to enhanced research about the incidence, control, and prevention of mental illness.

ICD-10 Specifics

The WHO's ICD-10, with the US adaptations (ICD-10-CM), was formally adopted in the USA on October 1, 2015. The USA maintains a naming convention for their classification and procedural system: ICD-10-CM and

ICD-10-PCS. PCS stands for Procedural Coding System, a system that has some impact on the behavioral health industry but will not be addressed extensively in this text. This transition from ICD-9 to ICD-10 was monumental for the healthcare industry and involved a large learning curve. Providers were anxious about the transition because of its foreseen disruption to the clinical landscape, due to the significant differences between the two systems.

The ICD-10 is dramatically different from its predecessor, the ICD-9. The sheer number of available diagnoses (approximately 68,000), documentation requirements, levels of specificity per diagnosis, and corresponding documentation requirements made the adaption of ICD-10-CM especially challenging. An easy-to-understand example of this is a "broken hand." In the ICD-9-CM, it was listed as a "closed fracture of the hand" but in the ICD-10-CM, it is listed as an "unspecified fracture of right wrist and hand, (initial for closed fracture)." Another example is for the diagnosis of Post-Traumatic Stress Disorder (PTSD). The ICD-9-CM listed one diagnosis for PTSD: 309.81 Post-Traumatic Stress Disorder. The ICD-10-CM lists three distinct PTSD diagnoses: F43.10 PTSD, Unspecified, F43.11 PTSD, Acute, and F43.12 PTSD, Chronic.

The USA had been using ICD-9-CM until this point and the shift from ICD-9-CM to ICD-10-CM can be further illustrated by Table 1.2:

Table 1.2 High-Level Differences Between the ICD-9 and ICD-10

ICD-9	ICD-10
Date WHO Approved: 1975	Date WHO Approved: 1990
Approximately 14,000 codes and diagnoses	Approximately 68,000 codes and diagnoses
Codes are 3–5 digits long	Codes are 3–7 digits long and alpha-numeric
2 Volumes, 17 Chapters	3 Volumes, 21 Chapters
Not very descriptive of diagnoses	Significantly more descriptive

The term "expansion" is commonly used when referring to the changes between the ICD-9-CM and the ICD-10-CM. In addition to the increase in the number of codes, the ways conditions are labeled, assessed, and documented are significantly more expansive. This expansion has been part of the challenge and pushback from providers about ICD-10-CM. The increased specificity of the codes necessitates far more comprehensive clinical documentation. These documentation requirements have become the focus of audits and compliance programs, which have been instated to ensure the new diagnoses have corresponding, supportive documentation.

The ICD-10-CM implementation was additionally complex because the codes themselves serve multiple purposes. Given that the USA does not have a single-payer healthcare system, many stakeholders rely on the ICD for claims, reimbursement, medical decision-making, documenting medical necessity, policies, and so on. The content of "what" goes into the ICD system in the USA is so important because the diagnoses work in conjunction with other stakeholder motives; more specifically, if a certain diagnosis is not listed in the itemization, then third-party payers will likely not reimburse providers for treating those conditions. Interest in the ICD-10-CM and the process for vetting diagnoses has even stirred controversy within the healthcare system.

The ICD-10-CM has 21 chapters (see Table 1.4, pp. 14–15). The ICD-10-CM codes will begin with an alpha character, followed by several digits. The alpha characters correspond with the chapter section of the ICD-10-CM covered by that grouping. For the Mental, Behavioral, and Neurodevelopmental Disorders, which are found in Chapter 5 of the ICD-10, the alpha-character assigned is "F." The subsequent characters in the code will represent:

- The *Diagnosis Category, digits two and three*: Drug-of-Choice or Conditions such as Alcohol, Major Depression, Anxiety;
- The last four digits represent: the *etiology, severity, and manifestation* of the disorder, with the very last digit being a possible placeholder for additional information.

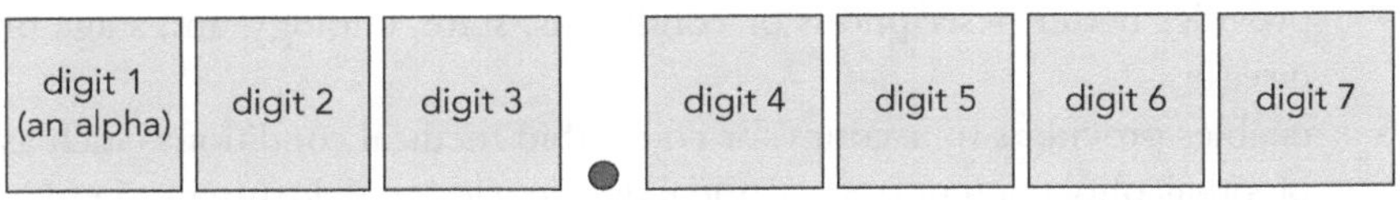

More specifically:

- **Digit 1**: This will be an alpha character and will correlate to the chapter in the ICD-10-CM. Some examples of alpha prefixes are:
    - F = Mental and Behavioral Disorders, located in Chapter 5
    - X = Self-Harm codes, located in Chapter 20
    - Z = Additional codes that may be a part of the clinical picture, factors that influence health status, Chapter 21
    - T = Poisoning codes, Chapter 19
    - R = Suicidal, Homicidal Ideation codes, Chapter 18
    - E = Endocrine, Nutritional, and Metabolic Disorders, Chapter 4

- **Digits 2 and 3**: These digits represent the condition or drug of choice. For example:
    - 33 represents Major Depression, Recurrent
    - 10 represents Alcohol
    - 40 represents Anxiety
- **Digits 4–7**: These digits represent the etiology, severity, and manifestation of the diagnosis. There is an additional box that may contain a "placeholder" digit to allow for future expansion or additional information depending on the diagnosis and category (i.e. initial versus subsequent encounters).

Some Select Examples of ICD-10-CM Codes from ICD-10-CM Tabular List of Diseases and Injuries

As you can see from Table 1.3 the ICD-10-CM codes may seem overwhelming, but while they may seem overwhelming in scope and variety, the benefits of the ICD-10-CM far outweigh the challenges. By utilizing the ICD-10-CM coding system, healthcare providers can utilize a naming and coding system that:

- is more accurate and specific;
- provides better descriptions of conditions, state, etiology, and stage of disease;
- enables providers to account for co-morbid medical conditions (such as blood-alcohol content or nutritional deficiencies) and document them in a way that clearly conveys this diagnostic information to the client's other healthcare providers;
- provides a uniform tool to document with clarity what is actually transpiring with a client;
- holds clinicians accountable for treating specific conditions, not general broad-based conditions where the medical necessity is difficult to determine;
- enables research and statistics regarding population health to be more specific.

In addition to the benefits outlined above, behavioral health clinicians now have a way of diagnosing and communicating critical client conditions in discrete data elements such as a recent suicide attempt/ideation or other

Table 1.3 Samples of Code Formats in the ICD-10-CM Tabular Index

Chapter 5: The Mental, Behavioral, and Neurodevelopmental Disorders	
F10.251	Alcohol dependence with alcohol-induced psychotic disorder with hallucinations
F20.0	Paranoid schizophrenia
F30.12	Manic episode without psychotic symptoms, moderate
F43.12	Post-traumatic stress disorder, chronic
F55.1	Abuse of herbal or folk remedies
F73	Profound intellectual disabilities

Chapter 20: External Causes of Morbidity, Intentional Self-Harm Section, Purposely Self-inflicted Injury, Suicide (attempted)	
X73.0	Intentional self-harm by shotgun discharge
X78.1	Intentional self-harm by knife
X81.1	Intentional self-harm by jumping or lying in front of a (subway) train

Chapter 21: Factors Influencing Health Status and Contact with Health Services	
Z73.1	Type A behavior pattern
Z72.820	Sleep deprivation
Z71.52	Counseling for family member of drug abuser
Z69.010	Encounter for mental health services for victim of parental child abuse

Other Common Conditions Encountered During the Service Delivery of Behavioral Health Conditions, found in other ICD-10-CM Chapters	
E08-E13	Diabetes mellitus
I10-I15	Hypertensive diseases
I-26-I28	Pulmonary heart disease and diseases of pulmonary circulation
J44.9	Chronic obstructive pulmonary disease, unspecified
J45	Asthma

complicating factors that color the clinical picture. In the era of health information exchange, this specific articulation is imperative because all that might be communicated to other care providers is a select data set or itemization of the current diagnoses and/or medications. This feature, by itself, can be life-saving as mentioned.

ICD-10-CM codes, compared to their predecessors, provide far greater detail on the nature of the reported condition. The detail within these codes allows for the differentiation and delineation of risk and severity. Some of the additional attributes of conditions in many ICD-10-CM codes include:

- co-morbidities
- manifestations
- etiology / causation
- complications
- detailed anatomical location
- sequelae
- degree of functional impairment
- biologic and chemical agents
- phase / stage
- lateralization and localization
- procedure-related issues.

One concept from above to explicate further is lateralization and localization. Most of the ICD-10-CM codes also provide far more detail in order to increase specificity. The implication for behavioral health and substance use is that documentation now encourages specification for the location of self-harm and details necessary to support the diagnoses. The utilization of the X-codes, Intentional Self-Harm, is critical in behavioral healthcare. Despite working with suicidal clients, most behavioral health clinicians are unaware of the existence of these codes in the ICD-10-CM and why it is critical to use them. By using X-codes, we will be able to track increasing severity in the methods of self-harm, possibly alerting us to a pattern that could eventually have fatal consequences. If we are able to detect this pattern by tracking the diagnoses given (assuming the clinician has diagnosed the X-codes when appropriate), then we can intervene in clinically appropriate ways before a tragedy happens.

Behavioral health and substance use providers using ICD-10-CM now assign high-level medical conditions alongside behavioral health diagnoses, therefore accounting for other conditions and factors, which influence a patient's mental health condition, as well as abuse and neglect codes. Previously in the USA, medical conditions were noted in the narrative portion of the medical record, or assigned to Axis III in the DSM-IV-TR. These options will now require specific assignment of a corresponding code. This inclusion of medical diagnoses indicates a tremendous shift in clinical case formulation and conceptualization for most behavioral health providers. It can also be perceived as an uncomfortable shift from simply notating co-morbid medical conditions in the diagnostic summary to actually assigning a (medical) diagnosis code. The assignment of actual medical diagnostic codes will be addressed in Chapters 3 and 6.

Additionally, the ICD system provides healthcare practitioners worldwide with a common language, data set and comprehensive method of communicating the challenges clients encounter in a succinct, standardized manner. This standardization enables the collection of public health statistics, incidence rates, and other important information for research purposes. For example, a 2016 article published in *European Psychiatry*, the journal of the European Psychiatric Association, "The validity and reliability of the diagnosis of hyperkinetic disorders in the Danish Psychiatric Central Research Registry," looks at the incidence of diagnosing Hyperkinetic Disorder (i.e. known in the USA as Attention-Deficit Hyperactivity Disorder) according to the ICD-10 diagnostic criteria. Country-specific language differences aside, it is clear that having one set of clinical diagnostic criteria is critical for worldwide research purposes. In this case, the diagnostic classification system used is the *ICD-10 Clinical Descriptions and Diagnostic Guidelines*, also known as the "Blue Book." Most clinicians in the USA are not aware there is another diagnostic manual that corresponds to the ICD-10 codes, *The ICD-10 Classification of Mental and Behavioral Disorders: Clinical Descriptions and Diagnostic Guidelines* (ICD-10 CDDG). This manual will be discussed later in the chapter.

The ICD-10 is the current classification system published by the WHO. The ICD-11 Beta Draft version is currently open-source and available for review, comment, and feedback. It is hoped that after the Beta phase of the ICD-11 revision is complete, it will be presented to the World Health Assembly in 2018 for formal approval. For more information about the Beta phase of ICD-11, please see: www.who.int/classifications/icd/revision/en/.

The ICD-10-CM Tabular List of Diseases and Injuries, aka "The Tabular Index"

We have learned the basic structure and format for the ICD-10 codes. We have also learned that the codes contained in the ICD-10 are numerous, specific, and number close to 68,000. How exactly are the codes organized in the ICD-10-CM and will behavioral health clinicians need to know all 68,000 codes? The answer is that we need to know where to find *all the codes that pertain to providing our clients' care*, not just the mental and behavioral health codes. Many IT systems or reference materials distributed to staff in behavioral health settings are NOT inclusive of the entire ICD-10-CM code set. Rather, many resources contain only the codes that have been determined (by someone) to be important for diagnosing your clients, which is arbitrary and subjective.

It is important to understand the many "sources" available to obtain ICD-10-CM codes. Examples of these sources include, but are not limited to: the Internet, the DSM, and your Electronic Health Record (EHR), to name a few. While these options can be helpful, it is vital to understand that *these sources may not be exhaustive or precise*. To be certain, the single, authoritative source for ICD-10-CM codes in America is a CDC publication called the *ICD-10-CM Tabular List of Diseases and Injuries*, also known as the "Tabular Index." It is updated twice a year. Each year, a new version of the Tabular Index is published and made available to the public, free of charge.

Key Considerations

- The Tabular Index, published by CMS and the CDC, is the official listing of all the approved ICD-10-CM codes in the USA.
- This does not mean other resources are wrong, but it is ultimately the diagnosing clinician's responsibility to ensure the diagnosis code assigned is accurate and the most specific one available.

For those of you familiar with the coding industry, you will likely know that there are actually two indices, the Alphabetic Index and the Tabular Index. These indices, and the rationale for focusing on the Tabular Index will be addressed in Chapter 3.

The Tabular Index itemizes the diagnoses and codes and remains the only validated, HIPAA-compliant, and definitive itemization of diagnoses and codes. It is each clinician's responsibility to not only know the source of the codes and diagnoses they use, but to also validate them against the Tabular Index for accuracy.

Behavioral health entities are very concerned with privacy and security of confidential information. Privacy, confidentiality, and regulatory requirements all govern how we disclose information. 42 CFR Part 2, which is being revised for the first time in decades (at the time of this writing), will give us better guidance regarding confidentiality parameters. Clinicians must also adhere to HIPAA. HIPAA discusses privacy and security matters, and it may be surprising to learn that HIPAA also informs us what guidelines to use when coding, documenting, and reporting in the healthcare record. Specifically,

"HIPAA-Compliant" Code Sets

The notion that the ICD-10-CM is the only "HIPAA-complaint" code set to be used in electronic healthcare transactions has been difficult to understand for those in the behavioral health industry. There is some controversy regarding this statement as well. To understand this, we must go back to the conversation, "Are these DSM codes or ICD codes?" Since the numerical values are identical in many cases, what is the difference?

- Correct: numbers and numerical values are indeed the same as long as the code assigned is the correct ICD-10-CM code. Regardless of the source for the code number, there is no problem with compliance if it can be validated by the ICD-10-CM Tabular Index.

  - Example: F33.3 in the DSM-5 is "Major Depression, Recurrent Episode With Psychotic Features" (DSM pg. 162). F33.3 in the Tabular Index is also "Major Depression, Recurrent Episode with Psychotic Features." This is considered a one-to-one match.
  - Important note: The American Psychiatric Association (APA) did attempt to select the best ICD-10-CM corresponding code for the DSM-5 diagnoses, yet no version of "crosswalks" are perfect. The APA has indicated that the ICD-10-CM code in parenthesis in the DSM-5 manual is indeed an ICD-10-CM code.

- Healthcare claims in the USA are largely submitted electronically to third-party payers. There is a place on these claims to itemize the diagnosis(es) treated for that particular healthcare encounter. *This space on the claim must only contain a HIPAA-compliant, industry standard code value from the ICD series.*
- Electronic healthcare claims must meet National Standards for Electronic Data Interchange (EDI) published by the American National Standards Institute (ANSI).
- HIPAA requires the use of "X12 standardized transactions" on all electronic transmissions that contain Protected Health Information (PHI). Electronic submissions must also use Version 5010 for compliance with federal law.
- Per HIPAA, Covered Entities must use the ANSI-approved, X12 standards and only the ICD-10-CM codes have been approved for these EDI transactions (not the "DSM codes").

74 FR 3228, the HIPAA Administrative Simplification Rule published January 16, 2009, Section IV A, states that *all HIPAA-covered entities must follow the ICD-10-CM Official Guidelines for Coding and Reporting*. The Coding and Reporting Guidelines will be thoroughly addressed in Chapter 2.

The Tabular Index is updated twice a year as a result of ICD-10-CM Coordination and Maintenance Committee meetings. This index can be found on the CDC's website and is located in a zip file on the homepage for the ICD-10. Under the heading "FY 201X Release of the ICD-10-CM" you will see an option to download the ICD-10-CM in PDF format. Contained in that zip file are five indices: Drug, E-Index, Index, Neoplasm, and Tabular. You will pick the "Tabular" to download the 1,910 pages of the 2017 ICD-10-CM codes that are currently recognized and authenticated.

The Tabular Index is a free, open-sourced, and authoritative itemization of the ICD-10-CM codes for clinicians in the behavioral healthcare industry. It is also employed to validate whether other sources of ICD-10-CM codes are accurate. The Tabular Index has 21 chapters, delineates approximately 68,000 codes and covers all areas of medical and other health conditions. Chapter 5 of the Tabular Index is dedicated to the Mental, Behavioral and Neurodevelopmental Disorders (the F-codes), as we have discussed. The majority of work in the behavioral health industry will involve utilization of Chapter 5, the F-codes, but we will need diagnoses and codes from other sections of the Tabular Index as well. Table 1.4 illustrates the Tabular Index outline:

Table 1.4 The 2017 ICD-10-CM Tabular Index Table of Contents

The 2017 ICD-10-CM Tabular List of Diseases and Injuries		
Chapter	**Category/Condition**	**Code Block Number**
1	Certain infectious and parasitic diseases	A00-B99
2	Neoplasms	C00-D49
3	Diseases of the blood and blood-forming organs and certain disorders involving the immune mechanism	D50-D89
4	Endocrine, nutritional and metabolic diseases	E00-E89
5	Mental, behavioral and neurodevelopmental disorders	F01-F99
6	Diseases of the nervous system	G00-G99
7	Diseases of the eye and adnexa	H00-H59
8	Diseases of the ear and mastoid process	H60-H95
9	Diseases of the circulatory system	I00-I99
10	Diseases of the respiratory system	J00-J99

The 2017 ICD-10-CM Tabular List of Diseases and Injuries		
Chapter	**Category/Condition**	**Code Block Number**
11	Diseases of the digestive system	K00-K95
12	Diseases of the skin and subcutaneous tissue	L00-L99
13	Diseases of the musculoskeletal system and connective tissue	M00-M99
14	Diseases of the genitourinary system	N00-N99
15	Pregnancy, childbirth and the puerperium	O00-O9A
16	Certain conditions originating in the perinatal period	P00-P96
17	Congenital malformations, deformations and chromosomal abnormalities	Q00-Q99
18	Symptoms, signs and abnormal clinical and laboratory findings, not elsewhere classified	R00-R99
19	Injury, poisoning and certain other consequences of external causes	S00-T88
20	External causes of morbidity	V00-Y99
21	Factors influencing health status and contact with health services	Z00-Z99

Each chapter outlines the available diagnoses and code numbers approved by the CDC and used by the American healthcare industry. The Tabular Index, once downloaded from the CDC, is an invaluable resource, and it is recommended that you have a copy of it easily accessible.

Utilization of the ICD in America's Behavioral Health System

Despite the fact that the ICD-9-CM has been around for decades, it has been the DSM series that has been almost exclusively used by clinicians in the behavioral healthcare field in the USA. Clinicians in behavioral health have used the DSM series as their go-to manual for helping them conceptualize, formulate, and define problems to begin the process of treatment planning. The DSM series is a reference book that virtually every clinician in the industry in the USA has been trained on and has utilized. The awareness in the USA that there was another coding or diagnostic system available was virtually non-existent. Shifting to the ICD series in the USA is a large cultural change in the industry, yet so critical for population health and research purposes.

Starting in October 2015, all healthcare providers in the USA were mandated to implement the ICD-10-CM. This mandate includes behavioral health clinicians who were used to using the DSM series. Until then, virtually the only frame of reference for diagnosing, coding, and documenting mental health conditions in America had been the DSM series. Clinicians would utilize the current volume of the DSM to assess their client's symptoms, choose the diagnostic category, then assign diagnoses and code numbers from the DSM manual (see Chapter 4 for details on diagnosing per the DSM).

Code numbers are not only used for assigning a diagnosis to a patient. Code numbers serve multiple purposes; they:

- document that a healthcare service was delivered;
- provide the basis for planning care for the client;
- are placed in the client's medical record as the determination of the client's diagnosis;
- go on the claim form that is sent to third-party entities for payment processing;
- are used to determine medical necessity for treatment purposes;
- are used to communicate a client's condition to another care provider;
- help measure the safety, quality, and efficacy of medical care;
- could be used to determine legal disability status for benefits;
- are used to recognize and identify abusive or fraudulent reimbursement practices and trends;
- could be used for any number of other reasons including research, public health statistics, disease process monitoring, population health, and incidence reporting.

If you asked behavioral health clinicians how they assign diagnoses and what code numbers they use, the typical response you will hear is "We use the DSM codes, of course!" (In fact, this very comment was made by a participant on a clinical training course on ICD-10 and DSM-5 conducted by the author in Northern Virginia on May 5, 2016.) There is frequent confusion about "code numbers" in use between the ICD and DSM. The issue is whether or not the DSM has its own "code numbers" or if the code numbers itemized in the DSM-series publications are, in reality, ICD codes. The answer is that the DSM series has put the ICD code numbers into their publications but it has not been made definitely clear to the clinician that the numbers they *visually* see in the book are ICD code numbers. This is why clinicians *will say* they use DSM codes, not ICD codes. And while this has been true historically and did not pose a problem prior to October 2015 in the USA, the landscape became far more complex when the new DSM-5 was published in May 2013 and the ICD-10-CM came into effect.

While much of the USA is currently utilizing the DSM-5, some state agencies, Medicaid, and other entities have not yet transitioned to the new DSM-5. Instead, they continue to use the older version, the DSM-IV-TR. Implementing any new system is difficult for technological reasons, and there has been considerable debate as to whether or not we must use or transition to the DSM-5. The upshot is that a provider entity should use whichever DSM-version the regulatory and other third-party entity wants you to use at that given point in time. This could also mean that one third party will request information in the DSM-IV-TR format (i.e. all five Axes including a Global Assessment of Functioning or GAF score) while another third party may request clinical documentation and diagnosing using the new DSM-5 or ICD-10-CM (which has no Axes). Simply put, clinicians in our industry may be using different coding and classification systems concurrently in their day-to-day work, and these systems are not aligned in their diagnostic criteria or code numbers.

The ICD-9-CM has been used in the USA since 1979. DSM-IV was published in 1994. ICD-9-CM and DSM-IV have co-existed for a long time. ICD-9-CM code numbers, and the previously-used DSM series (DSM-IV-TR) have aligned with each other in the mental health section in about 98% of cases. Therefore, when a clinician looked in the DSM-IV-TR manual for a code number and picked a "DSM code," they were actually utilizing an ICD-9-CM code number. Table 1.5 gives us a clear picture of this issue:

Table 1.5 Sample Alignment of ICD-9-CM and DSM-IV-TR

DSM-IV-TR Descriptor	DSM-IV-TR Code Number	ICD-9-CM Descriptor	ICD-9-CM Code Descriptor
Depressive Disorder NOS	311	Depressive NEC	311
Anxiety Disorder NOS	300.00	Anxiety State	300.00
Schizoid Personality Disorder	301.20	Schizoid Personality	301.20
Anorexia Nervosa	307.1	Anorexia Nervosa	307.1

Most clinicians therefore had little idea they were actually using ICD-9-CM code numbers because their primary source had actually been the DSM manual. In fact, very few clinicians in the industry have understood this concept and that is partially why the transition to the ICD-10-CM created so much confusion in the behavioral health industry in the USA.

The industry at large got its first introduction to a potential conflict when the new DSM-5 was published in May 2013. The update from DSM-IV-TR to the DSM-5 had been developing for a long time and that process was quite controversial. Concurrent to the development of the DSM-5 was the awareness that the USA would have to transition to the ICD-10-CM at some point in the near future. The DSM-5 authors and contributors were aware of this transition and therefore went to great lengths to align the new DSM-5 code numbers with the proposed ICD-10-CM code numbers.

The DSM-5 is quite different than its predecessors (see Chapter 4). In the DSM-5, there are new diagnoses as well as new ways of conceptualizing diagnoses. In looking at the ICD-10-CM and the DSM-5, *different code numbers can be assigned to the same diagnosis, creating discrepancies that may have clinical implications*. See Table 1.6:

Table 1.6 Differences Between Systems Regarding F41.0 Code Number

F41.0 in the ICD-10-CM	F41.0 in the DSM-5
Panic Disorder without Agoraphobia	Panic Disorder

Please note that the F41.0 code number and corresponding description per manual were current as of the time of writing.

You will also find:

- Some diagnoses exist in the DSM-5 that are not present in the ICD-10-CM.
- There are diagnoses in the ICD-10-CM that are not in the DSM-5.
- The ICD-10-CM is much more specific in assigning “states” and code number digits to certain conditions (e.g. states = chronic, acute, and unspecified).
- The ICD-10-CM retains the familiar DSM-IV-TR diagnoses, structure, and classification for most behavioral and mental disorders, most notably the Schizophrenia and Substance Use sections.
- The DSM-5 has dramatically shifted these same categories of Schizophrenia and Substance Use, and so the discrepancies between the two systems are confounding to clinicians.

To its credit, the DSM-5 is a relevant predecessor to the eventual release of the ICD-11 by the WHO. The ICD-11 is currently being revised, with an anticipated release date sometime after 2018. At that time, it is projected that discrepancies between the ICD and the DSM will be far less significant, although still present. It is important to note, however, that the DSM is not the only diagnostic manual classification available, and its utilization varies from country to country. In fact, the DSM has been utilized by only a minority of psychiatrists worldwide, most notably in Europe where they use the Blue Book.

It is beyond the scope of this book to discuss the different available mental health diagnostic classification systems. Later in this chapter, however, we will discuss the available ICD-10 version of clinical descriptions and diagnostic guidelines that is used worldwide by those in the behavioral health sciences. But it is clear that in America there is an inherent tension between the utilization of the DSM and ICD series.

To summarize this section:

- Most professionals in the behavioral health industry in the USA have learned, utilized, and been mandated to use the DSM series as their main diagnostic, coding, and assessment tool for a variety of reasons, including: reimbursement, medical necessity, documentation of the delivery of services, legal status, etc.
- The DSM series is recognized in the USA as one of the manuals for determining diagnoses, codes, and assessment outcomes in the behavioral health industry.
- For third-party purposes, including HIPAA, reimbursement, and legal medical record-keeping, the ICD series is recognized by US government entities as the official diagnostic coding classification system.
- Some third parties still require the utilization of the DSM series concurrent to assigning an ICD-10-CM diagnostic code to the presenting problem.
- The discrepancies between the DSM and ICD series create problems for clinicians and consumers alike.
- Many providers in the behavioral sciences worldwide exclusively use the ICD series.

Cross-Referencing Code Sets: "Crosswalks"

We know that clinicians in the behavioral health industry in the USA will have different experiences with the various code sets required by different entities. We also know that various third parties, or stakeholders, will require utilization of different code sets at different times, for different reasons. This dynamic is similar to the concept of different payers requiring different elements to justify medical necessity for treatment being proposed during utilization reviews or for pre-certifications prior to the onset of treatment services. Jokingly, it has been said, *"Have five different payers? You will likely have five different requirements, sets of forms, and thresholds to meet! Good luck keeping it all straight!*" Table 1.7 illustrates this point:

Table 1.7 The Challenges of Using Multiple, but Required, Systems

Clinical Documentation for Payers; Utilization Review Requirements	Diagnosis Code Required on the Healthcare Claim
Prior authorizations may require all five Axes, or,	Per HIPAA, only ICD-10-CM codes are allowed on claims
Prior authorizations require ICD-10-CM diagnoses only, but also ask for a GAF score (Axis V), or,	Per HIPAA, only ICD-10-CM codes are allowed on claims
Utilization reviewers want DSM-IV-TR diagnoses, not DSM-5 diagnoses for substance use disorders, and yet they want DSM-5 diagnoses for all other conditions	Per HIPAA, only ICD-10-CM codes are allowed on claims

How do we get from one code set to another code set? How has the conversion from the ICD-9-CM to the ICD-10-CM taken place in a way to be so confounding to clinicians? Remember the ICD-9 had about 14,000 codes in it whereas the ICD-10 has approximately 68,000 diagnosis codes. This discrepancy is significant, as is the confusion.

While the most effective way of cross-referencing code sets is *to avoid* cross-referencing code sets, attempts have been made to help the clinician shift from a familiar code set to the new one. The terminology used and typical end product for this process has been labeled "crosswalks." It is very common to hear a request such as, "Do you have access to an ICD-9-CM to ICD-10-CM crosswalk?" Online websites and other technology advances have also helped facilitate this conversion, but this attempt to "clarify" can also be problematic (see the EHR section later in Chapter 1). While crosswalks can facilitate a clinician's hunt for the *approximate* location of a code, the precise code chosen needs to be made with old-fashioned clinical judgment: your brain. Let us look at why this is the case.

No crosswalk is 100% guaranteed for accuracy. Even the CMS General Equivalence Mappings (GEMs) Crosswalks carry a disclaimer that, in the end, it is the provider's responsibility to assign the correct diagnostic code. If not utilized properly, crosswalks can be a liability; now we are being asked to find code numbers that not only look unfamiliar, but also translate into different diagnoses than before.

The DSM-series proponents have mapped the DSM-5 codes to ICD-10-CM so the clinician does not have to search for the correct ICD-10-CM codes. While the intent was to be helpful, this mapping in reality is nothing more than another clinician's judgment as to which DSM codes align to ICD codes. It is important to note that some DSM-5 mappings frequently lead to "Unspecified" ICD-10-CM diagnoses and this will put everyone at risk if this particular crosswalk is solely relied upon. Further, there are some inherent problems and distinctions between the manuals, notably the presence of Substance Use, Abuse, and Dependence in the ICD-10-CM versus Substance-Use and Substance-Induced categories only in the DSM-5.

Table 1.8 illustrates a crosswalk and shows how diagnoses mutate across code sets. In addition to the different names and numbers of the disorders, keep in mind there are also different clinical criteria across code sets. (See the next section on the DSM and the Clinical Descriptions and Diagnostic Guidelines, or CDDG.) Table 1.8 shows how a diagnosis can change across the sets:

Table 1.8 How Diagnoses "Mutate" Across Systems

DSM-IV-TR	ICD-9-CM	ICD-10-CM	DSM-5
300.16: Factitious disorder with predominantly psychological signs and symptoms	300.16: Factitious disorder with predominantly psychological signs and symptoms	F68.11: Factitious disorder with predominantly psychological signs and symptoms ICD-10 also has: F68.12 & F68.13	NO DSM-5 DIAGNOSIS code F68.11 Closest is: F68.10: Factitious Disorder
315.1: Mathematics disorder	315.1: Mathematics disorder	F81.2: Mathematics disorder	F81.2: Specific learning disorder: with impairment in mathematics
333.7: Neuroleptic-induced acute dystonia	333.72: Acute dystonia due to drugs	G24.02: Drug-induced acute dystonia	G24.02: Medication-induced acute dystonia

Table 1.8 demonstrates a "one-to-one" match, meaning there is one code in one set that correlates to one code in another classification system. While the terminology across the sets may change slightly causing some confusion or documentation challenges, the intent of the code and diagnosis is to be categorized as one-to-one. These one-to-one matches are fairly straightforward, easy, and intuitive.

However, with 14,000 ICD-9 codes compared to 68,000 in the ICD-10, the majority of diagnoses will not have a one-to-one match. Rather, they will have a ratio of "one-to-many" and the ratio numbers can be as high as 1:3 (e.g. PTSD, Anorexia, Conversion Disorders) or 1:7 (e.g. Phobias and Schizophrenias). Another way of conceptualizing these ratios is to discuss ICD-10-CM in terms of "expansion." The ICD-10-CM is significantly more expansive in certain diagnostic categories than its predecessor, the ICD-9-CM. This phenomenon also applies to the DSM series as well, with DSM-5 being much more expansive than the DSM-IV-TR.

The categories of Substance Use, Anxiety, and the Bipolar diagnoses have the most expansion in them across the code sets. We will take a closer look at some of the differences in each diagnostic category in Chapter 4. The Substance Use category itself is especially expansive:

Table 1.9 Number of Substance Use Diagnoses in the DSM-5 versus the ICD-10-CM

DSM-5: Codes and # of Diagnoses	DESCRIPTION (ICD-10-CM) by Substance	ICD-10-CM OPTIONS: Codes and # of Diagnoses
F10s: 8	Alcohol	F10s: 47
F11s: 10	Opioids	F11s: 41
F12s: 10	Cannabis	F12s: 34
F13s: 8	Sedative, hypnotic, or anxiolytics	F13s: 52
F14s: 10	Cocaine	F14s: 44
F15s: 10	Other stimulants	F15s: 45
F16s: 8	Hallucinogens	F16s: 38
F17s: 4	Nicotine	F17s: 20
F18s: 6	Inhalants	F18s: 37
F19s: 7	Other psychoactive substance related disorders	F19s: 57

Clinical Descriptions and Diagnostic Manuals: The DSM and CDDG

Until now, we have been discussing the issue of ICD versus DSM diagnoses and the assigned code numbers. We will take a closer look at the code number differences in Chapter 4. The other important aspect of choosing a diagnosis or code number has to do with the clinical descriptions. Clinical descriptions are the typical characterizations or manifestations of certain health conditions. Usually, these clinical descriptions will describe and define the symptoms, clinical presentations, states, and severity of the patient's presenting problems in an effort to help the clinician assign the corresponding diagnosis. Once the diagnostic label is chosen, the corresponding code number is then referenced.

At a high level, the process for assigning a code number to a diagnosis in the behavioral health industry typically is as follows:

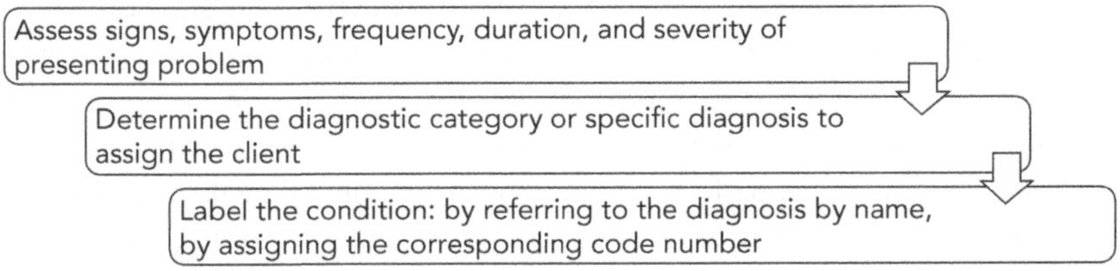

Note that the process of assigning and coding diagnoses generally differs between the behavioral health industry and the medical industry in America. This difference will be discussed in detail in Chapter 2.

For diagnostic accuracy, a clinician will refer to the clinical descriptions in a manual of their choosing. Currently in the USA, most clinicians turn to the DSM series for clinical descriptions and criteria. The WHO has also published an open-source manual of clinical descriptions that serves the same purpose: *The ICD-10 Classification of Mental and Behavioral Disorders: Clinical Descriptions and Diagnostic Guidelines*, also known as the ICD-10 CDDG. This publication, largely used outside of the USA, is intended for "general clinical, educational and service use." There is a different publication used for research purposes, the *Diagnostic Criteria for Research* (DCR-10). The DCR-10 outlines the research criteria to be used with the ICD-10 when studying mental and behavioral disorders. There are express instructions for how to use the DCR-10 in the beginning of the manual under "Notes for Users." The other manual, the ICD-10 CDDG, is sometimes referred to as the "Blue Book" because of the color of the cover and because of the URL for the free, online PDF version of the book. The research version is sometimes referred to as the "Green Book" for the same reason. It is the Blue Book that will be exclusively referenced and utilized in this textbook since clinicians use it the most. Researchers or other interested individuals can access the Green Book from the WHO (see Bibliography for details of the website).

In Europe, and in other areas of the world, many clinicians turn to the Blue Book to obtain their criteria for diagnosing a client with a mental, behavioral, or substance use condition. Even in 2016, the predominant diagnostic classification system used in Europe is the Blue Book. But in the USA, we have almost exclusively used the DSM series. In fact, medical necessity, medical policies, and admissions criteria are, for now, largely based on the DSM series. This may be in part due to the fact that there are no viable, up-to-date, current alternatives to the DSM since the Blue Book was last published in 1992. This will change when the ICD-11 is put into production and the ICD-10 CDDG will be updated to the ICD-11 CDDG, hopefully very soon after 2018. However, it is important to keep in mind that, on a global level, there is currently mixed utilization of both the DSM and the ICD clinical descriptions and criteria.

To illustrate the fact that the ICD and its clinical descriptions are driven by international forces (i.e. those that are not DSM-centric), let us look at the demographics of the WHO's Global Clinical Practice Network, or GCP Network. This is a group of approximately 12,600 mental health and primary care professionals from across the world who are contributing content and descriptions to the new ICD-11 CDDG. Membership numbers in 2016 include: 1,791 from the USA, 4,682 from Europe, 3,055 from the Western Pacific and Asia, and 1,399 from South America. One fundamental premise in this book is to propose that all behavioral health clinicians utilize the same manual, the ICD manual. The rationale for this involves globalization, interoperability, standardization, consistency, research, population health, and epidemiology purposes. Using the DSM sets the USA apart from the rest of the world. Arguably, which is better: using a manual that is influenced by limited interest groups and largely limited to one country, or using a clinical criteria manual that is developed in an open, transparent, and internationally cooperative manner?

There are clear and important differences between the DSM series and the Blue Book. Generally speaking, the Blue Book gives far more latitude to the diagnosing clinician to determine when a client meets the criteria for a certain condition. Contrast this with the DSM series where you will find concrete, time-limited, and frequency-specific itemizations of symptoms. Certain conditions in the DSM are also time-limited and the parameters for diagnosing such conditions can be interpreted in a strict sense by a variety of stakeholders. The reasons for the specificity of the DSM usage might be considered as follows:

1. The American healthcare system has been a fee-for-service system but is rapidly changing to require payment for services tied to both value and quality metrics. As a result, it is easier to grasp conditions that are clearly defined, even having starting and ending points.

2. The majority of the clinicians using the DSM series are not psychiatrists and therefore may need additional guidance as to when a client meets the threshold for the diagnosis.

It has been said that by using the Blue Book, the clinician is given latitude to *"practice the art of diagnosing"* whereas clinicians who may not be as experienced may need clearer operational criteria of when a diagnostic threshold is met. Apparently, this is one of the reasons why European psychiatrists *"absolutely love the Blue Book!"* However, just the presence of two different diagnostic classification manuals is problematic for the industry worldwide. It is because of this fact that one fundamental premise of this book (mentioned above) is to argue for the use of one, standardized, international diagnostic classification system: the ICD series. Indeed, the DSM is not inclusive of all the conditions or diagnoses that affect the behavioral health population. Using a system that is inclusive of diagnosing intentional self-harm, abuse, and neglect is imperative for the industry. The only comprehensive system that enables this is the ICD system.

The Blue Book is in the process of being updated to reflect the new codes and diagnoses that have been included since the inception of the ICD-10 in the 1990s. *The ICD-10 Classification of Mental and Behavioral Disorders: Clinical Descriptions and Diagnostic Guidelines* (CDDG) is undergoing a revision by the WHO that is intended to bring it into alignment with the upcoming ICD-11, around 2018. It will contain updated and current clinical descriptions, criteria, diagnoses, and conceptualizations of how certain conditions manifest, in order to ensure accurate assessment and diagnosing. This revision will give the clinician a viable, well-respected, free alternative to the DSM that is intended to complement the ICD-11 and that will enable clinicians to be consistent with all resource materials. As a matter of fact, the proposed ICD-11 CDDG will be quite sufficient to support the mental and behavioral disorders in the ICD-11. As a result, some say that the DSM series will be, or should be, rendered unnecessary.

To create the updated ICD-11 CDDG, international working groups were recruited and asked to collect diagnostic information that they encountered in actual practice. The working groups gathered and submitted this information to the WHO's Department of Mental Health and Substance Abuse Division. The information has been submitted utilizing "content forms" which are standardized templates in order to maintain a robust, consistent format for each clinical description. These standardized content forms will help provide the technical, clinical, and administrative information that will serve as the basis for the new ICD-11 CDDG.

The ICD-11 and corresponding ICD-11 CDDG are truly exciting, innovative, collaborative, and worldwide works of art. There is a wealth of knowledge on an international level with experts in behavioral health sectors who are actively working on the ICD-11 development. The ICD-11 is open-sourced, meaning all resources pertaining to the ICD-11 will be available worldwide, free of charge and readily available on the Internet or in other format to anyone who wants them. One of the concerns with the new DSM-5 has been the potential conflict of interest accusations regarding the pharmaceutical industry's influence on which diagnoses are retained (or not) in the new DSM-5.

Finally, the DSM series itself, as well as its digital version that many EHR vendors purchased to embed into their systems for end users' convenience can be cost prohibitive. Further the APA's digital DSM-5 limits the number of diagnoses available to clinicians by *only including the diagnoses itemized in the DSM-5*, which does not promote true integrated care service delivery or give access to critical self-harm and medical diagnoses. Therefore, having a truly collaborative international, comprehensive, and standardized set of reference materials (the ICD-11 and ICD-11 CDDG taken together) will be an exceptional advantage for public health and disease-incidence tracking, worldwide.

Concurrent Use of the ICD and DSM

In the US behavioral healthcare system, we are presented with the challenge of using two distinct diagnostic classification systems. This challenge presents options, but it also presents potential confusion. While there is considerable effort to harmonize these two systems, they will likely never be truly compatible. The behavioral health industry in America is the *only* healthcare industry *required* to utilize two different manuals and this complexity leaves the clinician in a position of having to study and know both systems to be truly adherent and compliant to each system.

US clinicians are also somewhat at the mercy of the regulators, governing bodies, licensing boards, and insurance companies. Every stakeholder may choose to utilize certain criteria or manuals, hinging reimbursement or payment for services based on their guidelines for medical necessity, "billable versus non-billable" diagnostic codes, or other discretionary guidelines. As mentioned earlier, clinicians will need to know the differences between the manuals and be prepared to utilize whatever classification system or diagnostic criteria guidelines an outside entity requires.

ICD-10-CM Contrasted to the DSM-5

Clinical differences between the ICD and the DSM series will be discussed in Chapter 4. As part of the contextual understanding of the relationship between the ICD and the DSM, a few points of difference should be addressed:

- The number of coded diagnoses is different. For example, there are approximately 415 Substance Use codes in the ICD-10-CM (the DSM-5 has approximately 81 with code numbers).
- The diagnostic and clinical criteria in the DSM-5 are different from the criteria used in the ICD-10 CDDG.
- The differences between the ICD-10-CM and the DSM-5 in the category of Schizophrenia are notable. The DSM-5 has one single coded diagnosis for Schizophrenia: "Schizophrenia Unspecified, F20.9" whereas the ICD-10-CM has several coded schizophrenia differential diagnoses. This is problematic for EHRs, clinical decision support rules, computer logic, client safety, and lab check alerts. Until this is rectified, it will remain problematic.
- Another major difference between the DSM-5 and ICD-10-CM is the entire category of Substance Use. The DSM-5 applies diagnoses labels of "Substance Use" or "Substance-Induced" whereas the ICD-10-CM uses the diagnostic terminology of Abuse or Dependence.
- An organization's EHR system obtains their ICD-10-CM codes from an outside entity. If the DSM-5 codes from the APA were embedded in the code tables of that EHR, this could lead to erroneous mappings that may be not be accurate and could create liability and fiscal concerns for the clinician and organization.

Devotion to the DSM series runs deep in America. Yet the mandate to fully utilize and implement the ICD series presents the clinician with conflicting challenges. It would be very forward-thinking for any stakeholder to make the determination to utilize only one system in the USA, namely the ICD series. It is expected that someday this uniformity will be the case in the USA.

Electronic Health Records and Mental Health Codes

Health Information Technology (HIT) has transformed the way healthcare is delivered across the globe. While the behavioral health industry is considered somewhat "behind" in its adoption and utilization of EHRs, clinicians will likely encounter EHRs in their jobs at some point. It is beyond the scope of this book to discuss EHRs at length, but it is imperative for behavioral health clinicians to understand how diagnostic codes function in an EHR. This is important because, most of the time, it is the direct service clinician who is ultimately responsible for assigning the most accurate diagnosis to their client at the point of service, not a coding department (see Chapter 2).

Most clinicians do not question the origin of the diagnosis codes in their EHR system. However, this process is automated and someone else has streamlined this cross-referencing for the clinician. Streamlining this process can lead to improper diagnoses and perhaps even imprecise care.

EHR vendors—the companies who sell you the EHR and are responsible for its development and maintenance—have obtained their diagnostic codes from a variety of sources. Among these sources are:

- private companies who employ certified coders to "crosswalk" the codes;
- private companies who have entire divisions devoted to coding;
- computer programmers who load the codes into the system;
- CMS GEMS mappings;
- the digital version of the codes in the DSM-5 from the APA.

While each one of these methods has its pros and cons, the bottom line is that it is the responsibility of the diagnosing clinician to ascertain that the correct diagnosis is made and documented in the client's legal health record. EHR vendors have not been forthcoming with the sources of the ICD-10-CM Behavioral and Mental Health codes in their systems. Additionally, one must be very careful because if certain of the methods above are used, the end user will not have access to the entire set of diagnoses in the ICD-10-CM, possibly creating unintended consequences such as claim denials or missed opportunities to diagnose for self-harm or medical conditions.

For example: we know that documenting suicidal and homicidal ideation is critical for a mental health record for a variety of reasons. Suicidality and Homicidal Ideation have typically been documented in the text-narrative portion of the client's record. If clinicians go back and read this text-narrative portion of the record, they will see the history of suicidal or homicidal ideation. If the clinician only looks at the page in the EHR that itemizes the diagnoses, and *if* suicidal or homicidal ideation are *not* diagnosed and coded in the EHR, then this critical piece of information will be missed. Many clinicians, and EHR vendors, are not aware that suicidal and homicidal ideation carries its own diagnosis codes (R-codes) in the ICD system. For so many purposes, it is essential to include all the available diagnoses in the EHR: computers report on discrete data sets, not on the narrative portion of the medical record. If it was not diagnosed, it may not be considered as existing if a report or CCD document does not pick it up.

Some EHR vendors are using sources for their "available ICD codes" from a limited data set, one that does not include the R-chapter codes where the suicidal and homicidal codes live. This does not just apply to some R-codes; this is applicable for medical codes, stressor or contributing factor codes, or any other codes/diagnoses that may be applicable to our client's current condition. In the past, these diagnoses were written out in the format of the DSM-series five Axes. But now that there are no more Axes in the DSM-5, how then would we document *and* diagnose what had been considered important correlating diagnoses such as Personality Disorders (Axis II), Medical Conditions (Axis III), and Stressors (Axis IV)?

Keep in mind that there are perfectly legitimate codes in the ICD-10-CM that are not contained in the DSM-5. Clinicians must utilize *all applicable codes* pertinent to devise a treatment record and plan based on a client's condition. This includes not only the applicable behavioral health diagnoses, but medical, self-harm, psychosocial, and other factors that influence a client's health status. The US Federal Office of Disease Prevention and Health Promotion (with its "Healthy People 2020 Campaign"), the Affordable Care Act, Certified Community Behavioral Health Centers and all other healthcare initiatives and reforms clearly emphasize addressing a person's entire set of healthcare needs. To do this, we must have access to and use *all applicable, appropriate ICD-10-CM codes*.

Regarding client safety, there can be significant risks in not utilizing all applicable ICD-10-CM codes. The following scenario will exemplify this point and highlight the concern about the source of diagnosis codes in your EHR:

Class Discussion

Let's say you are working with a client diagnosed with Paranoid Schizophrenia, in an outpatient setting. Since there is one variety of Schizophrenia in the DSM-5, the DSM-5 available diagnosis for this is F20.9, Schizophrenia, Unspecified. However, there is an ICD-10-CM code for Paranoid Schizophrenia, F20.0. If your EHR vendor uses DSM-5's electronic, recommended mapped code to ICD-10 CM for Schizophrenia (F20.9), you will then be assigning a ICD-10 CM code of "Schizophrenia, Unspecified."

The negative implications in this case are:

- The use of unspecified codes puts the provider at (financial and other) risk for not assigning the most specific code available to them per the ICD-10-CM Coding and Documentation Guidelines.
- The provider is unable to assign the *correct* diagnosis, Paranoid Schizophrenia (F20.0) if your vendor used only the DSM-5 digital version of the codes.
- Public health statistics and analytics are impacted.
- Clinical decision supports or alerts, including those for lab work or medications, may not be able to be leveraged within the EHR.

How might this be problematic? What else can you think of that might be challenging to you as a clinician?

Complicating variables in this process involve the way codes and diagnostic names are displayed in the actual EHR. How an end user searches for the codes, and which code-set "button" they may click on to obtain the drop-down itemization for that particular diagnostic category can be problematic. Some EHRs have individual code-set buttons (ICD-9, ICD-10, DSM-IV-TR, DSM-5). Others have "mapped" options such as "DSM-IV-TR to ICD-10-CM" to be helpful.

Options for Searching for Codes in an EHR

Term-based

Using one word, or part of a word to produce the diagnosis listing. This particular item is notable in that the language differences between clinicians and code sets can be quite problematic. For example, a clinician may search for "depression" but only a medical code for depression comes up (e.g. nose depression). However, if you type in "depressive" you will get a whole set of diagnoses that are more applicable. This option requires a thorough assessment of the system's diagnostic functionality prior to utilization (SNOMED CT can be helpful for this situation; see Chapter 5).

Search by Code

Search by code range, individual code numbers, or partial code numbers. This is a fairly reliable method of getting ICD-10-CM codes, provided we know the sourcing of the ICD-10-CM tables running in the background.

Alphabetical or Tabular-based

Search by the 2017 (or current year) Tabular Index or Alphabetic Index.

Concept-based

Similar to Term-based, but pulls tables from clinical concepts such as "depression" or "anxiety." This option also includes searching by SNOMED CT terms, which is the point of SNOMED CT (see Chapter 5).

Crosswalks

Search by the old ICD-9 code with results pulling ICD-10 suggestions, but it is important to know how any crosswalk was developed. This is not a reliable method for obtaining the ICD-10 codes and diagnoses.

Still others have other variations that can be confusing. Search options for codes and diagnoses also can present challenges: if a clinician searches for a term *"depressive"* versus *"depression,"* potentially a whole different set of available diagnoses will populate for the clinician to choose from.

Keep in mind that the technology *behind* these embedded codes is nothing more than computer-programmed code. Put another way, there is typically one code number per line item (e.g. imagine an Excel spreadsheet). Who puts what value into that cell (called "tables" in the EHR systems world) can make all the difference in giving a client a diagnosis of *"with psychosis"* versus *"without psychosis."*

Vendors are great at selling their products. They have been known to say, *"Don't worry about it. We have all the ICD-10-CM transition items taken care of for you in the EHR!"* This may not be the case at all. The reality is that clinicians have a new code set(s) to learn, and will be able to apply different diagnoses for items such as self-harm and diagnose and code for suicidal ideation in a way they have not before. And it is the responsibility of the clinician, not a computer system, to ensure the diagnosing is comprehensive and accurate.

Key considerations or questions to ask yourself and the EHR vendor are:

- How are your end users searching for the codes and is there a standardized way of doing this?
- What is your source of the ICD and DSM codes in the EHR?
- How will these codes be updated?
- What happens if all the available codes, such as Suicidal and Homicidal Ideation, are not available for use in the EHR?
- How will we know if the codes displayed are correct?
- Has your Quality Assurance or Medical Director validated the codes in the EHR with the ICD-10-CM Tabular List of Diseases and Injuries? Have they signed off that the codes embedded in the system are correct?

The answers to these questions will be dependent on the EHR vendor. Clinical leadership within each provider entity also bears responsibility to ensure accuracy of the ICD-10-CM codes in the EHR system. Decisions will need to be made about who is responsible for integrity of diagnosis codes in addition to how to actually assign a (medical) diagnosis to a client. Chapter 6 will address some of these organizational policy considerations for administrators and leadership to discuss.

Summary

1. The ICD system is a comprehensive diagnostic system for behavioral health clinicians to code all the conditions that affect our clientele, including critical diagnoses for intentional self-harm, physical health, and abuse/neglect conditions.
2. The only accurate protocol to assign a verified ICD-10 diagnosis is to reference the Tabular Index. Other references, such as "crosswalks," can be problematic for a variety of reasons.
3. It is recommended that clinicians use the clinical and diagnostic manual that aligns with the coded diagnoses recorded in the client's legal record. If this protocol is not followed, then the accuracy of certain diagnoses can be challenged (e.g. substance abuse and dependence in legal matters).

Bibliography

American Health Information Management Association. (2016). *ICD-10 FAQs*. Retrieved March 27, 2016 from www.ahima.org/topics/icd10/faqs.

American Psychiatric Association. (2016). *History of the DSM*. Retrieved March 27, 2016 from www.psychiatry.org/psychiatrists/practice/dsm/history-of-the-dsm.

Centers for Disease Control and Prevention. (2011). *International Classification of Diseases, Ninth Revision, Clinical Modification (ICD-9-CM)*. Retrieved May 16, 2016 from www.cdc.gov/nchs/icd/icd9cm.htm.

Centers for Medicare and Medicaid Services. (2016, January). *Billing Properly for Behavioral Health Services: Be Part of the Solution*. Retrieved July 8, 2016 from www.cms.gov/Medicare-Medicaid-Coordination/Fraud-Prevention/Medicaid-Integrity-Education/Downloads/behavior-billing-booklet.pdf.

CMS.gov. (2015, December 30). *ICD-10 Coordination and Maintenance Committee*. Retrieved March 27, 2016 from www.cms.gov/medicare/coding/icd9providerdiagnosticcodes/meetings.html.

Department of Health and Human Services. (2000). 45 CFR Parts 160 and 162, Health insurance reform: standards for electronic transactions; announcement of designated standard maintenance organizations; final rule and notice. *Federal Register, 65*(160). Retrieved March 27, 2016 from www.cms.gov/Regulations-and-Guidance/HIPAA-Administrative-Simplification/TransactionCodeSetsStands/Downloads/txfinal.pdf.

Department of Health and Human Services. (2009). 45 CFR Part 162, HIPAA administrative simplification: modifications to medical data code set standards to adopt ICD-10-CM and ICD-10-PCS. *Federal Registry, 74*(11). Retrieved March 27, 2016 from www.gpo.gov/fdsys/pkg/FR-2009-01-16/pdf/E9-743.pdf.

Govtrack.us. (2010, September 24). *Text of Rosa's Law.* Retrieved March 27, 2016 from www.govtrack.us/congress/bills/111/s2781/text.

Maj, M. (2014). EPA-1821–DSM-5, ICD-11 and the public image of psychiatry. *European Psychiatry, 29*(1), 1. DOI: http://dx.doi.org/10.1016/S0924-9338(14)78938-2.

Mohr-Jensen, C. et al. (2016). The validity and reliability of the diagnosis of hyperkinetic disorders in the Danish Psychiatric Central Research Registry. *European Psychiatry, 25*(16–24).

World Health Organization. (1992). *The ICD-10 Classification of Mental and Behavioral Disorders: Clinical Descriptions and Diagnostic Guidelines.* Geneva: World Health Organization.

World Health Organization. (1992). *The ICD-10 Classification of Mental and Behavioral Disorders: Diagnostic Criteria for Research*. Geneva: World Health Organization. Retrieved April 1, 2016 from www.who.int/classifications/icd/en/GRNBOOK.pdf.

World Health Organization. (2016). *International Classification of Diseases*. Retrieved March 27, 2016 from www.who.int/classifications/icd/en/.

2 The Coding and Documentation Standards

The topic of coding and documentation is minimally discussed in schools whose aim is to prepare graduate students for work in the behavioral health industry. The term "coding and documentation" is largely seen as a medical, financial, and reimbursement process for how medical records are created, maintained, and used for healthcare purposes. This chapter will explore the background for coding and documentation to further explicate the context and process by which the behavioral health industry has reached the point of necessary regulation and compliance to be true compatriots with the medical industry in the healthcare delivery system. This chapter will also explore the ways in which coding and documentation protocols apply to behavioral healthcare, documentation, diagnosis code assignment, data collection, and reimbursement. In addition, understanding the background of the coding and documentation standards will play a key role when we discuss ICD series compliance later in the book.

Over the past decades in America, we have seen a rise in documentation requirements, medical necessity criteria, and the general integrity of medical record-keeping in the behavioral health industry. While compliance is largely mandated by third party entities such as insurance companies and accreditation bureaus, it is equally important for the student to conceptualize that excellent documentation contributes to overall clinical competence. Currently, the quality of the behavioral health industry's records needs to correlate with the quality and documentation standards of our counterparts in the medical industry. AHIMA, the American Health Information Management Association, published a groundbreaking book, *Documentation and Reimbursement for Behavioral Health Services*. Unfortunately, many in the behavioral industry continue to assume that AHIMA relates only to the Health Informatics profession. In reality, AHIMA is a pertinent resource for practitioners in the behavioral field, and the standards set forth for documentation can, and should, easily extend to behavioral health settings. Lessons learned from this text could also set a gold standard for solid documentation.

However, the behavioral health industry has had a unique challenge: how do we notate and coordinate care around very sensitive information about mental illness and substance use / abuse in such a way that protects the consumer from harm? (For example: any reference in a medical record to a psychotic episode may be problematic for a high ranking senior management official if it becomes known and inadvertently disclosed.) Further, how do we balance the inherent tension between confidentiality and appeasing all the stakeholders in the healthcare industry, including the consumer, HIPAA, and third-party payers?

New delivery models of care, such as person-centered care, integrated health models, and recovery-oriented systems of care, require that the numerous professionals working with a single consumer can clearly, effectively and efficiently communicate with each other while simultaneously promoting client safety. In our current age of consumer care, behavioral health clinicians are working alongside many other healthcare disciplines as we treat the whole person (such as: medical, dental, case manager, and occupational and speech professionals), necessitating that we have a systemic, standardized way of managing the health information contained in a medical record. Increasingly, even the solo practitioner will likely be treating individuals who have other healthcare clinicians involved in their ongoing care, or who are required to exchange clinical information by participating in pay-for-value models. This coordination of care underscores the imperatives inherent in the healthcare field: to keep consumers safe and healthy, reduce readmissions, and reduce the morbidity of vulnerable populations with numerous co-occurring and compelling healthcare needs.

While programs to provide efficient and safe healthcare to consumers and to reduce recidivism rates have existed for years, several promising new models have emerged as of late. Each model identified below has one common component: coordinated, multidisciplinary healthcare delivery involved in treating the whole person; these include:

- Health Homes
- Patient-Centered Medical Homes
- Certified Community Behavioral Health Centers
- Accountable Care Organizations.

The current challenge in the health information technology sector, which impacts behavioral health clinicians, involves the Health Information Exchange mandates that are a part of the US healthcare programs as well as criteria for pay-for-value programs. Health Homes, for example, must be equipped to receive Continuity of Care Documents (CCDs) from other EHRs. As of this writing, there is still much work to be done in improving the "electronic disconnect" that exists in the healthcare system between EHRs. One of the premises of this book is that we need to truly begin to standardize the way we document and code for the conditions we encounter in our clinical settings. Having uniformity will facilitate improved quality care and population health in a way that utilizing two disparate systems (DSM and ICD) cannot.

As behavioral health clinicians and organizations, we must improve the way we have treated record-keeping and documentation if we plan to address the current healthcare quality problems in America. Specifically, we must share and be proficient in the healthcare language utilized by all healthcare providers involved in our client's care. Besides better care, this shared fluency in approach will move the healthcare dial toward overall population health.

The Institute for Healthcare Improvement (IHI) devised the "Triple Aim" to address healthcare quality concerns in the American healthcare system. The three components of the Triple Aim are:

1. improving the consumer experience of care (including quality and satisfaction)
2. improving the health of populations
3. reducing the per capita cost of healthcare.

Behavioral health clinicians play a critical role in helping achieve the Triple Aim. In order for us to contribute positively, we need to improve aspects of service delivery that have been long overlooked. Areas for improvement include: diagnostic coding, documentation, adherence to best and evidence-based practices, standardized practices, and above all, comprehensive, whole-person treatment, regardless of discipline.

While it is beyond the scope of this text to delve into the details about coding and documentation in the medical industry, it is important to highlight the following: how medical coding and documentation has evolved over time, its context and background, and how it relates to the behavioral healthcare field. Understanding this background also provides a framework for how best to communicate with the other healthcare providers involved in mutual consumer care. Behavioral health clinicians must learn how to speak the same language as other healthcare disciplines. While some have argued that this translates into "the medicalization of mental health," others have proposed that this standardization of language will elevate our status as key providers in consumer care.

As HIPAA-covered entities, we must follow the ICD-10-CM mandates regardless of third party relationships. However, it is unclear how many behavioral health practitioners really understand the background, content, and processes related to this mandate. This chapter will discuss coding and documentation as it applies to the ICD series and the federal mandates for regulatory compliance in behavioral healthcare. It will also address the need for behavioral health clinicians to be multidisciplinary in their conceptualization and documentation of clinical cases in order to coordinate best care with other providers. As behavioral healthcare clinicians who are moving with the industry toward whole-person care, we must achieve comfort with the assignment of medical diagnoses and assigning their applicable codes to our consumers.

Coding in the Medical Industry

Keeping good medical records is not only best practice: it is the law. As far back as the Social Security Act of 1902, the medical records mandate has been clear regarding documentation:

> (27) provide for agreements with every person or institution providing services under the State plan under which such person or institution agrees (A) *to keep such records as are necessary fully to disclose the extent of the services provided to individuals receiving assistance under the State plan*, and (B) to furnish the State agency or the Secretary with such information, regarding any payments claimed by such person or institution for providing services under the State plan, as the State agency or the Secretary may from time to time request.
>
> (Social Security Administration, Sec. 1902, 42 U.S.C. 1396a, Section 27. Emphasis added.)

At this time in the healthcare system, most medical entities use a software program called an encoder to assign the diagnostic code to a medical encounter, which is then submitted on the healthcare claim form. There are a variety of styles of encoders, but, for the most part, the encoder does the work of extracting out the billable codes and performing "claim edits" (i.e. ensuring that the codes on the claim forms are accurate, are not incompatible with other information on the form, and will most likely result in payment). An encoder is diagnostic and procedural coding, EHR-interfaced software, which contains computer-assisted coding, ICD-10-CM content, and clinical documentation improvement tools.

Consistent Language for Coding

The term "coding" is frequently used interchangeably with "codes." To clarify terms in this chapter, the following distinctions can be made:

Coding (by Provider or Clinician)	The actual assignment of a diagnosis code to a client's healthcare encounter, such as Depression, PTSD, Adjustment Disorder, Asthma, etc. **Inpatient Process**: The licensed provider responsible for the diagnosis is expected to document in such a way that the coding department personnel can assign the accurate diagnosis. **Outpatient Process**: The licensed provider may choose the diagnosis themselves and submit electronically, or use a manual paper process to choose the diagnosis they would like submitted to the third-party payer. Certified coders may also process outpatient services.
Coding (by CPC)	The process of reviewing a medical record/chart note and assigning the most specific diagnosis to the healthcare encounter. This applies to both inpatient and outpatient service delivery and may take place in a designated "Coding" or "Health Information" department.
Coding (by Encoder)	An encoder is a diagnostic and procedural coding, EHR-interfaced software program, which contains computer-assisted coding, ICD-10-CM content and clinical documentation improvement tools. These software systems help organizations by: 1. calculating an Inpatient Diagnostic Related Group (DRG), which is an inpatient payment rate 2. calculating an Outpatient Ambulatory Patient Classification (APC), which is an outpatient payment schedule 3. providing coders with coding guidelines and compliance, as built-in edits and references prompt accuracy.
CPT Codes	Current Procedural Terminology (CPT) codes are used to communicate what type of healthcare encounter took place. Examples include: 90791 (Diagnostic Evaluation), Health and Behavioral Codes, Evaluation and Management Codes. These are not the same as diagnosis codes!

Diagnosis Codes	The alpha-numerical ICD-10-CM value assigned to specific diagnoses to communicate a consumer's condition. Examples: F33.2 represents Major Depression Recurrent, Severe without psychotic features; Z69.010 represents Encounter for mental health service for victim of parental child abuse.

The traditional method of coding in the medical industry involved a medical coder (person) who read the record, extracted the information out of the record, and assigned the diagnoses to the healthcare encounter. Typically, coding and documentation in the medical industry will look similar to this process:

Inpatient Process

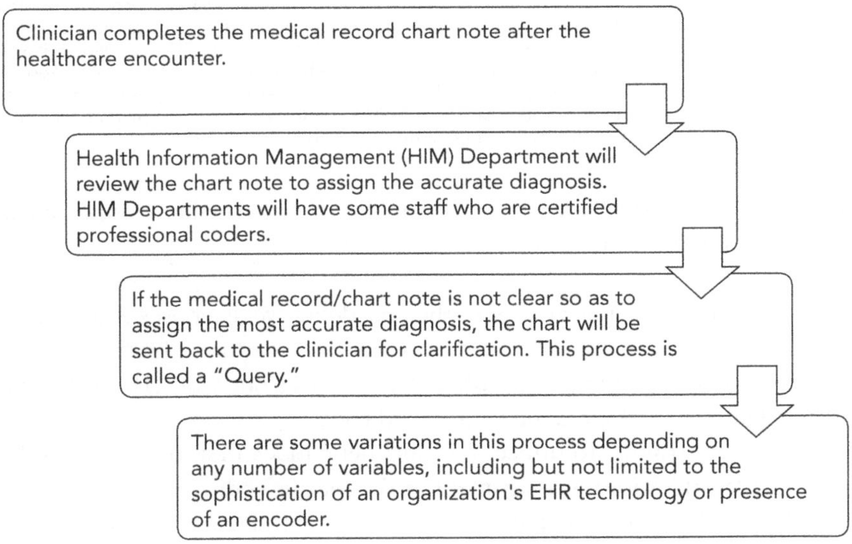

Outpatient Process

Each one of the above steps may have further variations depending on the organization or the robustness of the clinical technology solution. There can also be variations on the processes in the flowcharts above and it is up to each provider or organization to determine the process and flow that best fits the

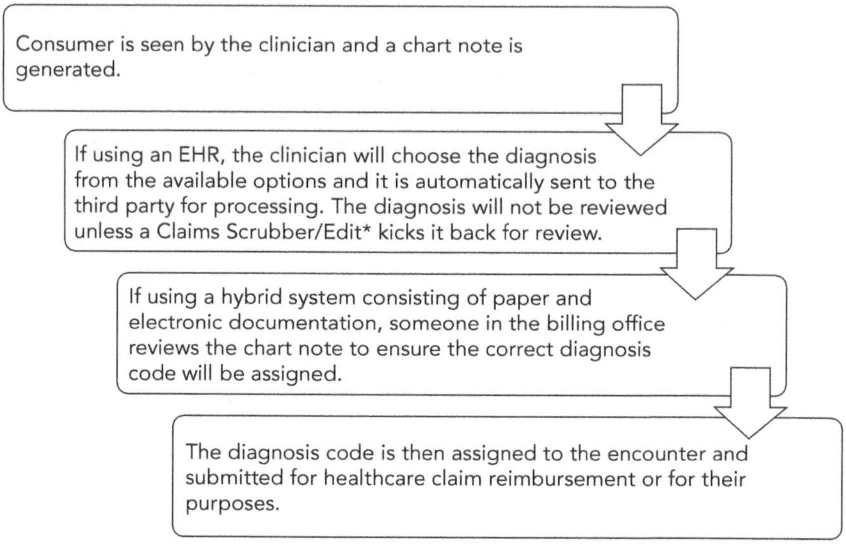

*Claims Scrubber/Edit: an automated electronic software program to verify that the code headed to the third party is legitimate and/or that it passes any number of pre-determined controls before being submitted. An example of a control is: any code that includes the work "Unspecified" in it may be kicked back for manual review to verify its accuracy. CMS has a number of rules, called "edits" regarding proper coding. The term "claims scrubber" is often used synonymously with "encoder" or "claim edits." Also, Health Information Management (HIM) staff may review any encoder flags and send these questions back to the clinician before the claims go out the door.

regulatory and compliance requirements for their particular circumstance. Some variations may include:

- The rendering clinician assigns the final definitive diagnoses and codes.
- The diagnosis name is written/typed out in its entirety by the clinician and the billing office (or Certified Professional Coder, CPC) looks up and assigns the corresponding ICD-10-CM code.
- CPCs are trained to utilize the Alphabetic Index first, then turn to the Tabular Index for the assignment of the specific code.
- A paper "superbill," charge master sheet, or itemization of billing codes, including CPT codes, may be handwritten by the clinician and submitted to the billing office.
- CPCs sometime use "encoders" (software programs) to help them find the diagnosis codes.
- There needs to be a line of communication between the provider and the professional coding staff when documentation does not support the most appropriate code assignment. There is a fine line between interpreting a provider's assigned diagnosis, reviewing the chart note, and the provider

perhaps having to amend the chart note via an addendum to clarify the encounter outcome for purposes of assigning a specific diagnosis.

In order for CPCs to assign the most specific, accurate diagnosis, they must rely on the clinician's chart note. One of the challenges with this is that if the chart note is not clear (for example: chronic versus acute exasperation of a condition), the clinician will have to be queried. A query is where the record is sent back to the clinician for clarification on the diagnosis to be assigned. This sometimes precipitates the clinician producing an addendum to the medical record; this whole process is resource-consuming, and creates inefficiencies. In essence, the specific documentation holds the key to assigning the diagnosis. Without specific documentation, a definitive diagnosis cannot be assigned. Previously, the ICD-9-CM system in the USA did not require the level of specificity that the ICD-10-CM now requires. The ICD-10-CM contains highly specific, very detailed diagnoses that require supporting documentation in order to substantiate the diagnosis assigned.

According to the Coding and Documentation Guidelines discussed later in this chapter, clinicians are highly encouraged to assign the most specific diagnosis code(s) available that are supported by the documentation. Unspecified codes are generally frowned upon. The CMS have indicated that if, during audits, they determine a code is not as specific as it could be, or if the documentation does not support the actual code assigned, then this could be a trigger for a payback, or, worse, an accusation of fraud or waste. Because the transition from ICD-9-CM to ICD-10-CM requires a higher level of specificity than ever before seen in the industry, CMS allowed providers some flexibility in the first year after implementation (through October 1, 2016). While not overtly denying codes with "Unspecified" diagnoses on them, it is likely that the utilization of Unspecified codes is being monitored and may put the provider at risk if a more specific diagnosis is available and warranted.

Coding in the Behavioral Health Industry

Before discussing coding in the behavioral health industry, we need to consider the following items:

- There has not been an industry standard for assigning codes and diagnoses.
- The utilization of certified coders in behavioral health settings is low, albeit growing, as more behavioral health settings employ CPCs and HIM professionals.

- Who actually assigns a diagnosis differs from entity to entity.
- Unless the clinician works in a typical medical setting, coding and documentation protocols are not usually followed.
- Most behavioral health clinicians have never heard of, let alone utilized, the Alphabetic or Tabular Indices.

A CPC will tell you that the only correct way of assigning diagnosis codes is to use the Alphabetic Index first, and then turn to the Tabular Index to assign the final diagnosis code. This is the formal and accepted process in the medical industry. Another fundamental premise of this book is:

> Behavioral health, in order to be treated as equal compatriots with the medical industry in the healthcare delivery system and who are bound by HIPAA, must begin to code and document like the rest of the healthcare industry. It is recognized by the authors of this book that asking behavioral health clinicians to use the Tabular Index, much less an Alphabetic Index *then* the Tabular Index, is highly unlikely to occur. Therefore, it is the recommendation to the behavioral health industry that *if we can just get clinicians used to verifying their assigned diagnosis codes in the Tabular Index AND follow the Coding and Documentation Guidelines,* this will bring us much closer to being compliant, adherent, and contributing to population health. This would be considered both industry-changing and a huge improvement!
>
> (Author's own words, 2015)

Outpatient Processes

The process for assigning diagnoses in the behavioral health industry can be different than assigning diagnoses in the medical industry. However, some behavioral health facilities that follow a traditional medical model—such as free-standing psychiatric hospitals, psychiatric units within acute care facilities, and outpatient behavioral health clinics affiliated with large medical entities such as the Mayo Clinic—have the infrastructure and processes in place to adhere to a more medical coding protocol. Interestingly, as the regulatory environment has become more stringent, many behavioral health organizations are starting to employ CPCs to assist in coding and documentation monitoring. We are beginning to see some of the more informal coding practices—typically found in outpatient behavioral healthcare—as targets for auditors and other regulators; as a result, organizations are becoming more proactive and scrupulous in securing comprehensive and accurate coding and documentation procedures.

For most outpatient behavioral health providers, the coding process looks like this:

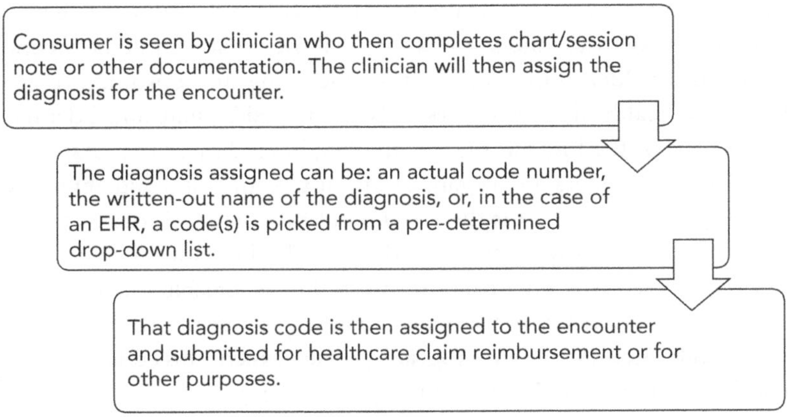

There is even greater variation in the behavioral health industry on the basic diagnosis coding workflow outlined above. Unfortunately, some of these variations can also put provider organizations at risk. An example of risk may include the following, erroneous diagnosing protocols:

1. Have the rendering clinician assign a DSM code to the encounter. This is then submitted to the billing office. The billing office, typically not comprised of CPCs, uses internally-generated references or crosswalks to assign the ICD-10-CM code to the claim. Sometimes the references used by the billing office are not verified as acceptable.
2. Have the billing office read the chart and assign the most appropriate ICD-10-CM code to the encounter (without a CPC's oversight).
3. In California, for example, the county-contractor provider organization submits a DSM diagnosis to the county after the service is rendered. The county, in turn, uses a CMS-approved crosswalk to submit an ICD diagnosis to Medi-Cal for reimbursement.
4. Handwritten encounter forms with CPT and diagnosis codes are supplied to the billing office. Billing office then types in the information on the healthcare claim form for submission.

While there is no single, unified process of behavioral health coding through to revenue cycle, some of the above variations could be problematic. One could argue that the variations above pose greater risk to clients receiving behavioral health diagnoses than the variations discussed in the medical industry.

Getting the laterality of a broken arm incorrect on a healthcare claim does not have as serious an impact as incorrectly assigning a mental illness diagnosis to a consumer. In most states, there are very clear regulations about who is authorized to assign mental health or substance use diagnoses. The process of assigning diagnoses, and who has control over that, should be a concern to every stakeholder in the organization, including the consumer. Assigning diagnoses to healthcare encounters is also regulated by state and federal laws.

The Office of the Inspector General (OIG) has indicated that "Assumption Coding" puts providers and organizations at risk for fraud and abuse. What is "Assumption Coding?" It is the assignment of a diagnosis or code without supporting clinical documentation in the record. There must be documented verification of services, and diagnosis, from the responsible provider in order to substantiate the diagnosis assigned. One way to ensure this is to have an active Quality Assurance (QA) program in place which runs coding audits and Clinical Documentation Improvement (CDI) programs.

Consider some of the following issues regarding the variations in Table 2.1:

Table 2.1 Coding and Documentation Scenarios, Myth and Risk Assessment

Scenario	Pros	Cons	Myth	Risk?
Rendering clinician assigns DSM code and billing office converts it into an ICD code	Saves clinician time Clinician does not need to be trained on ICD-series	Billing office personnel not CPCs DSM to ICD conversions are not all 1:1 Clinician is liable for billing office misdiagnoses Clinical judgment necessary, especially regarding substances	"This has worked in the past, so why won't it work now?" "If we are using a crosswalk, what difference does it make?" "The Internet has reliable sites for ICD conversions and obtaining the codes!"	Yes
Billing office personnel, not CPCs, assign the ICD code	Saves clinician time	Billing office personnel not CPC or trained to interpret medical charts Not licensed to assess and assign diagnoses Clinician is liable for misdiagnoses	"We have always done it this way." "I've been working in billing for 30 years and I know the codes." "As long as the insurance company sends us money, how can this be problematic?"	Yes

Scenario	Pros	Cons	Myth	Risk?
California: Submit DSM code to county; county uses CMS-approved crosswalk for Medi-Cal	Longstanding workflow	County personnel are not likely CPCs Entire medical record not going to the county, just a DSM-code DSM to ICD conversions are not all 1:1 Clinical judgment in converting DSM-ICD is necessary, especially regarding substances DSM-5 diagnoses in Substance Use category are not aligned with ICD-10 language	"This is the statewide system in CA so it must not be problematic." "Every county in CA uses the same crosswalk." "Trained personnel at the county are converting the diagnoses so I feel comfortable doing this."	Yes
Handwritten diagnosis codes sent to billing office for typed claim entry	Longstanding workflow	Poor handwriting, some guessing at the digit Human error with data entry	"The diagnosis is close enough to the right one." "Our clinicians won't do it any other way."	Yes

Where Does a Diagnosis Code Go? Lost in Translation

Unfortunately, most clinicians are not trained to understand where a diagnosis travels following the consumer encounter. Most behavioral health clinicians also likely assume that, when they assign a diagnosis to a client, it is that exact diagnosis that is placed on a healthcare claim form. Diagnosis codes can have serious and unintended consequences for all stakeholders. Clinicians may or may not know that insurance companies monitor the healthcare claims for all parties: they monitor utilization and trends coming from the clinician's office and they monitor and record the claim data for patient profiling. An easy example is a consumer with a history of suicide attempts who applies for a life insurance policy. Data repositories and patient profile histories may reveal this history and possibly lead to the underwriter of the insurer denying the application.

In previous versions of the DSM and ICD, where the diagnostic classification manuals and code numbers were aligned in most cases, thinking about diagnoses has not been a chief concern. Due to the seamlessness of the diagnosing process, clinicians had been lulled into a false sense of security. However, with ICD-10-CM and DSM-5 both concurrently in use, we encounter significant complications, in part due to the disparate classification systems, but also in terms of risk to the clinician. As long as there is utilization of the DSM and ICD concurrently, this will be problematic. Moving to a single consistent system, the ICD series, makes the most sense for integrated care service delivery and overall population health moving forward.

Let us look at two frequently-used diagnostic categories in the industry: Schizophrenia and Substance Use. The clinical differences between the manuals for these two categories will be discussed in Chapter 4.

To illustrate the problem with the diagnostic category Schizophrenia, the illustration below has been developed to outline the available diagnoses in the two manuals.

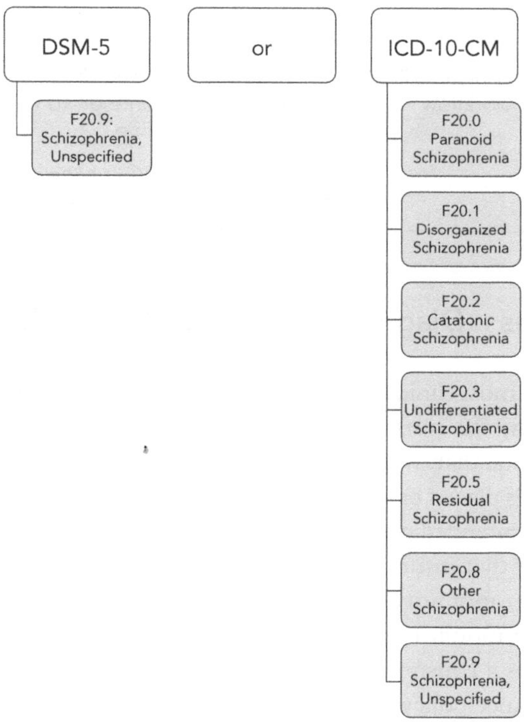

As you can see in the illustration, there is one variety of Schizophrenia in the DSM-5 manual. Yet the 2017 ICD-10-CM lists seven varieties of Schizophrenia (F20.8 is further subdivided into two more diagnoses). While this is straightforward in terms of which manual itemizes what, it becomes problematic when we look at some of the variations on how clinicians may assign diagnoses to clients. Here is one scenario, as an example:

California Psychologist Smith sees his client, Joe. Joe is known to be a longstanding Paranoid Schizophrenic. In the DSM-5, the only available code number is F20.9 Schizophrenia, Unspecified, and this is the code number Psychologist Smith must put on the form that he submits to the county. The county in turn submits F20.9 to Medi-Cal and Joe is now on record with the state as being an Unspecified Schizophrenic, instead of the most accurate diagnosis of ICD-10-CM: F20.0 Paranoid Schizophrenic.

- What are the implications for this scenario?
- How might this affect Joe?
- How might this affect Psychologist Smith?

Another major discrepancy between the DSM and ICD exists in regard to Substance Use categories. The language and diagnostic category differences create further problems, as seen in Table 2.2:

Table 2.2 Substance Use, High-Level Categories Demonstrating DSM-5 versus ICD-10-CM

DSM-5 Substance-Related Disorders	ICD-10 CM Mental and Behavioral Disorders Due To Psychoactive Substance Use
Substance-Use Disorders	Substance Use
Substance-Induced Disorders	Substance Abuse
	Substance Dependence

If you recall our California scenario, this situation is just as confounding as in Schizophrenia. While clinical differences will be discussed in Chapter 4, for now consider the following scenario:

- A clinician submits a required DSM-5 Substance Use diagnosis to the county: F10.20,"Alcohol Use Disorder, Moderate." The county then submits this code to the state as an ICD-10-CM code: F10.20, "Alcohol Dependence, uncomplicated."

- What are the implications for the consumer in this scenario?
- Is the client told that they have been diagnosed with a chemical "dependence" or a chemical "use disorder"?
- How might the therapeutic relationship be affected by this difference?

- Additional Note: F10.20 in the DSM-5 represents two different diagnoses: "Alcohol Use Disorder, **Moderate**" and "Alcohol Use Disorder, **Severe**."

  - When submitting just a code number, how is the distinction made between these two different diagnoses in a computer?

- What is the implication in California if the DSM-5 code number assigned and submitted to the county is intended to be Severe severity but the ICD-10-CM code sent to the state is instead just Moderate?

Free-standing psychiatric hospitals and other medical facilities which provide psychiatric care such as acute-care hospitals and emergency departments are not that much different in their coding processes than the medical industry workflow discussed earlier. There are a few considerations, however, that are particularly notable with psychiatric hospitals.

While inpatient psychiatric facilities typically have a coding department alongside the HIM and revenue cycle operations, the process for Admit-Discharge-Transfer (ADT) diagnosing is different than in an outpatient setting.

When a client presents to the inpatient psychiatric facility, an admitting attending physician (psychiatrist) will obtain enough basic clinical information to assign a high-level, typically "unspecified" diagnosis. Sometimes, the attending physician is securing clinical information over the phone by admission staff on site and giving admitting orders, while the clinical staff is documenting the official date and time of the orders and interacting with the client. The diagnosis given by the attending physician is then communicated to the client's insurer for pre-certification or by utilization review personnel.

Once the client is admitted, there is a typical amount of time allowed before a complete psychiatric evaluation must occur. At this point, the psychiatrist will likely revise the admitting diagnosis and assign a more comprehensive, specific diagnosis. The treatment plan for the patient's length of stay at the hospital and other orders will then be given.

Regarding inpatient diagnosing, it is highly recommended that, if a client's length-of-stay (LOS) is greater than 14 days, then the discharge diagnoses should be as specific as possible; the use of Unspecified should be used sparingly, if at all, and a clinical rationale should be documented. Auditors will monitor certain physicians and facilities to see if there are any trends of Unspecified diagnoses given after a 14-day LOS. The demarcation of 14 days is somewhat subjective and open to interpretation by various entities.

The CMS/CDC Coding and Reporting Standards: Overview

The majority of *behavioral health and substance use* provider entities in America have never learned the Official Guidelines for Coding and Reporting provided by the Centers for Medicare and Medicaid Services (CMS) and the National Center for Health Statistics (NCHS). Nor have providers been held consistently liable in a tiered chart review process to assess if their documentation does or does not meet a certain threshold of excellence. Therefore, there is a false and potentially dangerous assumption in the behavioral health industry that documentation is not important and that clinicians are not required to follow the documentation guidelines mandated by these regulatory bodies. It has also been reported that clinicians were never taught this information in their advanced educational programs. Leadership and administrations across the country have similarly not received adequate education and are also at this disadvantage. Establishing a systemic, standardized approach to thorough graduate school training will help organizations onboarding new employees and will minimize the amount of on-the-job training necessitated to maintain requirements and standards.

The document *ICD-10-CM Official Guidelines for Coding and Reporting FY 2017* is little known in our industry. Yet it contains much of the information necessary for an accurate and standardized approach to behavioral healthcare documentation objectives. In fact, utilization of these guidelines is mandated by HIPAA and is designed to:

> accompany and complement the official conventions and instructions provided within the ICD-10-CM itself . . . *Adherence to these guidelines when assigning ICD-10-CM diagnosis codes is required under the Health Insurance Portability and Accountability Act (HIPAA)*. The diagnosis codes (Tabular and Alphabetic Index) have been adopted under HIPAA *for all healthcare settings*.
>
> (Centers for Disease Control and Prevention, 2016, 1. Emphasis added.)

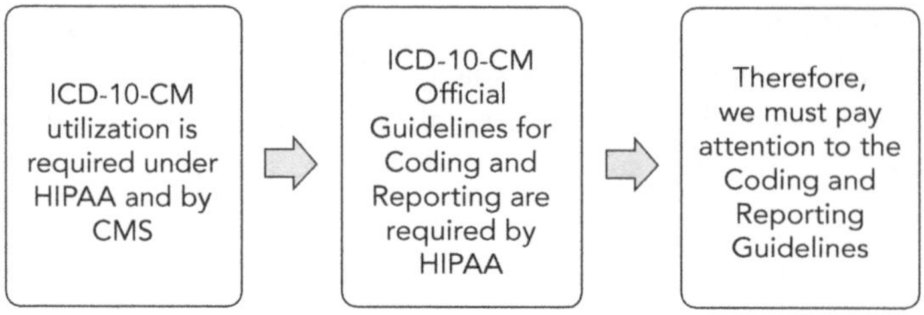

The chart above reflects the thought process and rationale for why we need to pay attention to the coding and reporting guidelines. In addition, third-party payers will typically enforce these guidelines, and ICD-10-CM compliance audits will also utilize these guidelines during reviews. The guidelines seem to be a new piece of information for practitioners. Yet, if one reviews the general conventions in the behavioral health industry for diagnosing and documenting they may recognize some of the guidelines already being implemented (just not formally). Even the American Psychiatric Association's (APA's) DSM-5, on page 23 of the manual, covertly endorses following the *"specific recording protocols for these diagnostic codes."*

The *ICD-10-CM Official Guidelines for Coding and Reporting FY 2017* is a free, 115-page PDF document that can be downloaded from the CMS ICD-10 website. It is a structured document that has been approved for use by the Cooperative Parties for the ICD-10-CM: the American Hospital Association (AHA), AHIMA, CMS, and NCHS. The table of contents is extensive and the document is easy to navigate from the table of contents by way of hyperlinks.

The rest of this chapter will take you through the mission-critical components of the guidelines document in a condensed, practical manner so you can both apply the conventions and guidelines for compliance per the regulations. Please keep in mind that these guidelines, although mandated, were written for those in the medical industry. There are many portions of the guidelines that are not applicable to behavioral health clinicians and these will not be discussed. The specific guidelines discussed are the ones determined to have the most impact on a community behavioral health center. If you are in another work setting, there may be other guidelines that apply to you. Best practice is to look at the guidelines yourself and determine what is applicable to your healthcare setting or business processes.

ICD-10-CM Guidelines for Coding and Reporting

Conventions

The first of two notable sections of the document gives the reader basic information about the standard approach to coding (i.e. diagnosing) and reporting. This Section I is titled, "Conventions, general coding guidelines and chapter-specific guidelines." Key elements for behavioral health clinicians are highlighted in this section to pay attention to and will be discussed separately below.

Conventions are the general rules for the ICD-10-CM that are to be used in addition to, or independent of, the actual guidelines. Among the conventions that are applicable to behavioral health in particular are:

1. The Alphabetic Index and Tabular List: This tells us that the ICD-10-CM is officially divided into the Alphabetic and Tabular List along with some other tables.
2. Format and Structure: ICD-10-CM code numbers have a standardized structure, including digits, alpha-characters, and numerical values.
3. Abbreviation Meanings: e.g. NEC stands for "Not Elsewhere Classified" and NOS stands for "Not Otherwise Specified."
4. "Code Also": This appears in the Tabular Index adjacent to a diagnosis if *two* codes are required to fully explain a presenting problem.
5. Other and Unspecified Codes: Defines these terms and when to use them.
6. Excludes Notes: Defines the utilization of these conventions.
7. "Code First": Defines how to apply these when there are co-morbid medical diagnoses.

Numbers 1–4 above are fairly straightforward and self-explanatory. However, numbers 5–7 need further explanation as they have a significant impact on the practice of behavioral health diagnosing.

Other and Unspecified Codes

This section clearly defines when we can use, or not use, diagnosis codes that contain the words "other" or "unspecified" in them. When we were utilizing the DSM-IV-TR and ICD-9-CM, these codes were labeled as NOS. However, in the DSM-5 the NOS designation has been replaced with Other Specified Disorder or Unspecified Disorder. Most instances of these types of designations in the ICD-10-CM are labeled as either "other" or "unspecified" diagnoses. Occasionally, you will see NEC in the Tabular Index. It is this particular guideline, coupled with the enhanced specificity in ICD-10-CM, that has created much confusion for US healthcare providers. The guidelines state the following:

> **Unspecified codes:** Codes titled "unspecified" *are for use when the information in the medical record is insufficient to assign a more specific code.* For those categories for which an unspecified code is not provided, the "other specified" code may represent both other and unspecified.
>
> **Other codes:** Codes titled "other" or "other specified" *are for use when the information in the medical record provides detail for which a specific code does not exist.* Alphabetic Index entries with NEC in the line designate "other" codes in the Tabular List. These Alphabetic Index entries represent specific disease entities for which no specific code exists so the term is included within an "other" code.
>
> (Centers for Disease Control and Prevention, 2016, 10. Emphasis added.)

In other words, Unspecified diagnoses should only be used when the information in the record does not support a more specific diagnosis or a more appropriate code does not exist. The box below shows an example of this.

> You do not get enough information during the Intake session to assign a specific Depression diagnosis so you choose "Depression, Unspecified."

Utilization of Other and Unspecified is not prohibited, but must be used under certain circumstances and not used exclusively, especially in long-term treatment cases. Overuse of Unspecified and Other places providers at risk for reimbursement paybacks because payers will require a specific diagnosis to help support the medical necessity threshold. While we are allowed to use these diagnostic designations, utilization of these diagnoses should:

- follow the ICD-10-CM Guidelines;
- have a clinical rationale, clearly documented in the chart, for why they are the best choice in any given situation;

- be supported by a clinical policy on utilization of Other and Unspecified diagnoses;
- preferably use the designation "other" with clear written documentation, rather than "unspecified," to mitigate risk during reviews and audits.

In fact, there is a specific guideline (to be discussed shortly) outlining the acceptable uses of Other and Unspecified.

Class Discussion

Discuss the pros and cons of using Unspecified or Other diagnoses. Give examples of times when Unspecified might be warranted or not. Finally, discuss the implications of *not* assigning an Unspecified diagnosis to a child. In other words, why might you want to use Unspecified for a child versus a more specific diagnosis?

Excludes Notes

Another coding and documentation guideline applicable to behavioral health is the "Excludes" rules. In the Tabular Index, you will find the terms "Excludes1" and "Excludes2." The illustration below outlines the formal definitions:

Excludes1: The codes excluded should not be used at the same time as the code above the Excludes1 note. Use when two conditions cannot occur together	Excludes2: Indicates the condition excluded is not part of the condition represented by the code. A patient CAN have two conditions at the same time

Excludes1 means you CANNOT diagnose certain conditions together at the same time while Excludes2 indicates that you CAN diagnose certain conditions concurrently. While a little challenging to understand because the terms appear to be counter-intuitive, it is best explained by examples:

- Excludes1: You CANNOT code/have a diagnosis of Amnesia NEC (R41.3) AND F44.0 Dissociative Amnesia at the same time; you CANNOT code/have R63.0 Loss of Appetite AND F50.0 Anorexia concurrently.
- Excludes2: You CAN diagnose an Adjustment Disorder AND Major

Depression at the same time; you CAN diagnose an Affective/Mood Disorder AND Separation Anxiety Disorder at the same time.

"Code First" (The Etiology/Manifestation Convention)

This convention is one of the more challenging coding rules we will encounter in the ICD-10-CM. Simply put, "Code First" means that certain conditions have an underlying cause (etiology) and a possible underlying manifestation due to the underlying etiology. This convention requires that the underlying cause be "sequenced" (listed/coded/diagnosed) first. It largely comes into play in the diagnostic categories of Substance Use, some Affective Disorders, and the cognitive disorders. This ICD-10 convention can be confounding for clinicians and their organizations.

The APA's DSM-5 talks explicitly about this convention on page 23 and acknowledges the existence of the ICD coding rule. The DSM recommendation is that practitioners diagnose the principal diagnosis/condition as the mental disorder "due to the medical condition," and then they are to list the medical disorder as the secondary diagnosis. The reason for the visit, or principal diagnosis, can then be followed by the qualifying phrase: "principal diagnosis." Yet, on page xiii, clinicians are instructed that "the code and name for the other medical condition should be listed first immediately before the mental disorder due to the medical condition."

Most behavioral health clinicians in the USA are not medical doctors. Counselors, social workers, psychologists, therapists, and drug and alcohol specialists typically do not have the medical training or scope of license to diagnose medical conditions. When discussing assigning an ICD-10-CM code to a medical condition, most behavioral health clinicians are not comfortable with the idea of assigning a diagnosis code to a medical condition.

This rule raises a number of considerations:

1. The DSM-IV-TR had five Axes. Axis III was slated to itemize medical conditions. Many clinicians did not hesitate to document co-morbid medical conditions such as Diabetes, Hypertension, or Immune Disorders. These were not given a coding-diagnosis number. Rather, the conditions were written out. If clinicians routinely did this with DSM-IV-TR then the question arises as to why behavioral health clinicians would not continue this practice with the ICD-10-CM? What is so different about writing out the name of the medical condition versus assigning a diagnosis code number to it?
2. Even some psychiatrists (who are medical doctors) are not comfortable distinguishing between the different types of medical conditions. For

example, there are numerous variations of Diabetes. Without being an endocrinologist, many psychiatrists are much more comfortable assigning a "high-level" Diabetes diagnosis to the case than a very specific diagnosis.

3. How do we handle integrated, holistic care models in which treating and tending to the medical condition carries as much relevance as helping our client with their mental health condition? What is the behavioral health clinicians part in assessing the medical condition and its impact on the mental health condition?
4. Regarding EHRs: if we put the medical condition in the *narrative* portion of the record because we are not comfortable assigning an actual diagnostic code to the medical condition, other providers who may receive a CCD may not be alerted to the client's complete diagnostic picture if medical diagnoses are not coded. This also applies to other providers who may have access to the client's record in the EHR, who may take a quick look at the Diagnosis tab only, but *not all diagnoses are itemized* as code numbers in the Diagnosis section of the record. This not only applies to the medical diagnoses but also to the X-codes which are the intentional self-harm codes.

Every clinician and organization may have a different approach to managing the "Code First" rule. Most important to consider are the scope of practice issues in your state, the push for whole-person care and the management of acute and chronic illnesses, and also the imperative to be mindful that the ICD-10 CDDG itemizes in its Annex frequently-encountered medical conditions in a psychiatric setting. Given the above-mentioned concerns, it seems necessary to code for and to diagnose medical conditions. The remaining question is how to code and document in a manner that is manageable by the provider and ensures quality care for the client.

The answer to this conundrum is twofold. First, implement a clinical policy and procedure that outlines how to code / diagnose the medical condition at a high level, as opposed to making a specific diagnosis. For instance, your organization may decide to code medical conditions to the third or fourth digit in an ICD-10-CM coding number instead of all the 6–7 digits that indicate a very specific diagnosis. You may have other ideas that work for you. Second, what remains imperative is for the clinicians to find a way to balance the "Code First" rule in congruence with complete client care and comprehensive medical documentation.

The Guidelines

After itemizing the conventions in the document, guidelines are then listed. Among the guidelines that are most pertinent to behavioral health clinicians are:

1. locating a code in the ICD-10-CM
2. level of detail in coding
3. use of Sign/Symptom/Unspecified codes.

Locating a Code in the ICD-10-CM

This guideline delineates how the medical industry conducts "diagnosis coding" by utilizing the medical record, CPCs and the coding or HIM department, the Alphabetic Index and then verifying the code in the Tabular Index. It gives us a very clear path to how we are to choose and assign ICD-10-CM diagnosis codes. It brings up the question, "Where do we get our ICD-10-CM diagnosis codes?"

For purposes of simplifying, standardizing, and streamlining the diagnosis code processes while adhering to the coding guidelines, it is recommended that all behavioral health clinicians use the current Tabular Index (discussed in Chapter 1) to verify the codes contained in their other manuals, EHRs, or reference materials when assigning diagnoses. While the Alphabetic Index is an important part of the coding processes, a licensed clinician who is comfortable assigning diagnoses should utilize the Tabular Index. Remember, the Tabular Index is the only official listing of acceptable, compliant diagnosis codes for utilization in the healthcare system.

Level of Detail in Coding

It is this particular guideline that concerns many in the US healthcare system. This guideline requires the clinician to assign the most specific diagnosis available to a consumer. Some diagnoses are listed first at a higher level, with subcategories or subdivisions listed underneath in the Tabular Index. Specifically, the guideline reads:

> Diagnosis codes are to be used and reported at their highest number of characters available.
>
> (Centers for Disease Control and Prevention, 2016, 14)

When looking at the Tabular Index, you will see how some diagnostic categories list one diagnosis whereas others list several under the main heading.

You will also note that the code numbers vary in length from 3-character to 7-character codes. The guideline indicates that we should use the most specific code, or subdivision, available to us. Typically, 3-character codes are category headings that may or may not be further subdivided. You are allowed to use a 3-character code *only if* it is not further subdivided. Finally, a code is considered invalid if it has not been coded to the fullest number of characters available.

Let us look at some examples to fully understand this particular guideline.

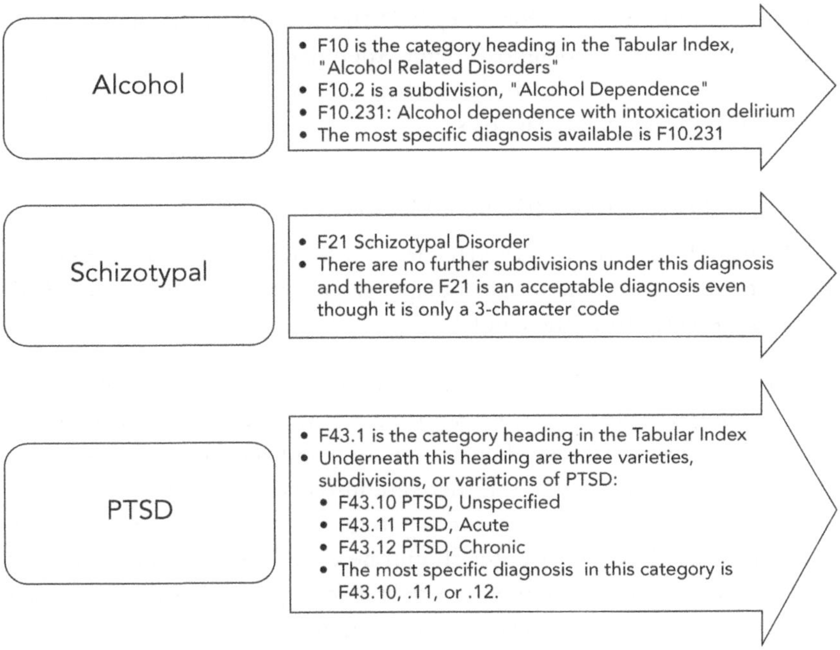

As you can see from the chart, 3-character codes tend to be category headings, and therefore not reportable diagnosis codes. Let us look at the diagnostic category of Alcohol: F10 only informs us that the problem being addressed is *Alcohol-related*, but we know nothing more than that. F10.2 indicates *alcohol dependence*, but this is still not specific enough for ICD-10-CM purposes. We have to drill down to the highest number of characters available to use in order to achieve the most specific, acceptable diagnosis code. F10.23 gets us to *Alcohol Dependence with Withdrawal*, but again, it may not specific enough. Finally, we get to F10.231, *Alcohol Dependence with Withdrawal Delirium* to achieve the highest degree of specificity in that category. It is this 6-digit code that the payers will likely require. Additionally, we must document in the record to substantiate each of the elements, or all necessary digits of the code chosen.

Let us look at the PTSD sample in terms of assigning the diagnosis code with the highest level of specificity. Your consumer will not just have a diagnosis of PTSD; they will have one of the three subdivisions of PTSD. And, of those three subdivisions, Unspecified can only be used according to the other conventions and guidelines. Practically speaking, if you have seen your consumer for any period of time, they will likely have either PTSD acute, or chronic, for the main diagnosis.

Finally, the documentation in the clinical note must support the most specific diagnosis used. One way to think about this is to consider making a documentation notation for every ICD-10-CM digit used; if there are five major keywords in the diagnosis name, then document to support each of those five elements. If this is done, then clearly your documentation will substantiate the assigned diagnosis.

Use of Sign/Symptom/Unspecified Codes

The final guideline to be discussed has to do with the utilization of Unspecified and when it is acceptable to use a diagnosis that is Unspecified. Here is the important excerpt from the Guideline:

> Unspecified codes have acceptable, even necessary, uses. While specific diagnosis codes should be reported when they are supported by the available medical record documentation and clinical knowledge of the patient's health condition, there are instances when unspecified codes are the best choices for accurately reflecting the healthcare encounter. Each healthcare encounter should be coded to the level of certainty known for that encounter. If a definitive diagnosis has not been established by the end of the encounter, it is appropriate to report codes for sign(s) and/or symptom(s) in lieu of a definitive diagnosis. When sufficient clinical information isn't known or available about a particular health condition to assign a more specific code, it is acceptable to report the appropriate "unspecified" code.
>
> (Centers for Disease Control and Prevention, 2016, 18)

The key to using Unspecified rests on the following important point:

- Use Unspecified if it is indeed the code that most accurately reflects what is known, and that is all the documentation supports, at the time of the healthcare encounter.

In behavioral health, it is often difficult to diagnose a consumer with a highly specific diagnosis until we have spent enough time with them. Some consumers are poor historians of their own mental health issues, and others may be reluctant to share information. Generally speaking, it would be important to have an internal clinical guideline about when and how Unspecified diagnoses are to be utilized at your place of practice. This will be discussed further in Chapter 6.

Chapter-Specific Guidelines

After the guidelines are delineated, the document moves on to discuss "Chapter-specific" guidelines. There are 21 chapters in the ICD-10-CM Tabular Index, each with its own guidance about how to code, diagnose, and document the conditions found within that chapter. Most attention will be spent on Chapter 5, the Mental, Behavioral, Neurodevelopmental Disorder chapter. Other chapters with guidelines pertinent to the practice of behavioral health will also be covered.

There is not a lot of Chapter-5-specific information in the document. In fact, there are only two diagnostic areas covered by Chapter 5: Pain Disorders and Substance Use. It is important that even though Pain Disorders appears to be a relatively low-incidence disorder, we will still discuss the guideline. Let us look at each diagnostic area.

ICD-10-CM Pain Disorders are located in the F45 category section of the Tabular Index. An example is "F45.41, Pain Disorder exclusively related to psychological factors." This is a subcategory of F45, Somatoform Disorders. The coding guideline states:

- Assign code F45.41 for *pain that is exclusively related to psychological disorders*. This is essentially a stand-alone diagnosis.
- F45.42, Pain disorders with related psychological factors should be used with a code from G89, Pain NEC if there is documentation of a psychological component (with acute or chronic pain).

(Centers for Disease Control and Prevention, 2016, 36)

Notice the word in *F45.41* of "exclusively." This means that clients presenting with somatoform pain will most likely be assigned this diagnosis. However, if you feel you have a consumer who meets the diagnosis for *F45.42*, the presence of the term "Code Also" present in the Tabular Index adjacent to this diagnosis, you must also notate a diagnosis of G89.xx which is a Pain Disorder diagnosis from Chapter 6, Diseases of the Nervous System.

Unless you work in a hospital setting, or intensive outpatient behavioral medicine facility that treats chronic pain, you will most likely encounter only *F45.41* in your day-to-day world.

When discussing the Substance Use section of the ICD-10-CM coding and documentation guidelines, remember that the only categories available for diagnosing are Use, Abuse and Dependence. This is, of course, different than the DSM-5. The Substance Use guidelines in the document can best be summarized in Table 2.3:

Table 2.3 Interpreting the Coding and Documentation Guidelines

Coding and Documentation Guideline states:	Interpretation/Comments
If you use an "in remission" code, this will be dependent on provider "clinical judgment." Also, the diagnosis code assigned must be supported by the provider documentation in the chart note.	You may obtain your diagnostic criteria for "in remission" from another manual, provided you have a standardized and consistent written policy for how you get to this diagnosis. Also, be clear in your documentation about the length of sobriety to support your standardized diagnoses.
If Use, Abuse and Dependence are present for the same substance, then diagnose according to a hierarchy. If use and abuse are present, code for abuse. If abuse and dependence are present, code for dependence. If all three are present, use dependence.	Again, there may be diagnostic criteria available to you that are helpful to make the distinction between categories. A shorthand way of remembering this guideline is to simply assign the more severe of the categories present.
The documentation for substances, and the relationship to any mental or behavioral disorder, should be clearly documented.	Make sure to delineate clearly in your diagnostic assessment the criteria on which you based your diagnosis in the ICD-10-CM.

In addition to the Chapter 5 guidelines, there are a number of guidelines for other conditions that will have an impact on the practice of behavioral health clinicians. Table 2.4 highlights the most important factors to consider when diagnosing and documenting for these conditions. Best practice is to review the entire coding and documentation guideline document and make decisions regarding what guidelines may impact your business processes. Table 2.4 itemizes all the other coding and documentation guidelines that impact behavioral health clinicians, and their interpretations for utilization:

Table 2.4 All Pertinent Coding and Documentation Guidelines for Behavioral Health

Item/ Condition	Coding and Documentation Guideline states:	Interpretation/ Comments
HIV	Code only for "confirmed" cases of HIV. In this context, "confirmation" does not require documentation of positive serology or culture; the provider's diagnostic statement that the patient is HIV positive, or has an HIV-related illness is sufficient.	Documenting and coding for HIV presents numerous challenges for behavioral health clinicians. Suggestion: Establish a clinical policy.
Poisoning	When coding a poisoning or reaction to the improper use of a medication (e.g. overdose, wrong substance given or taken in error, wrong route of administration), first assign the appropriate code from categories T36-T50. The poisoning codes have an associated intent as their 5 or 6 character (accidental, intentional self-harm, assault, and undetermined). Use additional code(s) for all manifestations of poisonings. If there is also a diagnosis of abuse or dependence of the substance, the abuse or dependence is assigned as an additional code.	This particular item will most likely be experienced when working in substance use or acute care facilities. Note the references to "intent" and the categories of use, abuse, and dependence. Also note the requirement to diagnose additionally abuse and dependence of the substance, if warranted.
Under Dosing	Under dosing refers to taking less of a medication than is prescribed by a provider or a manufacturer's instruction. For under dosing, assign the code from categories T36–T50 (fifth or sixth character "6"). Codes for under dosing should never be assigned as principal or first-listed codes. Non-compliance (Z91.12-, Z91.13-) or complication of care (Y63.6–63.9) codes are to be used with an under dosing code to indicate intent, if known.	This is a nice option to track medication non-compliance.
Toxic Effects	When a harmful substance is ingested or comes in contact with a person, this is classified as a toxic effect. The toxic effect codes are in categories T51–T65. Toxic effect codes have an associated intent: accidental, intentional self-harm, assault, and undetermined.	This will be helpful to document and code when there are intentional self-harm episodes.

Table 2.4 *continued*

Item/ Condition	Coding and Documentation Guideline states:	Interpretation/ Comments
Abuse and Neglect	Sequence first the appropriate code from categories T74.- (Adult and child abuse, neglect and other maltreatment, confirmed) or T76.- (Adult and child abuse, neglect and other maltreatment, suspected) for abuse, neglect and other maltreatment, followed by any accompanying mental health or injury code(s). If the documentation in the medical record states abuse or neglect, it is coded as confirmed (T74.-). It is coded as suspected if it is documented as suspected (T76.-). For cases of confirmed abuse or neglect an external cause code from the assault section (X92–Y08) should be added to identify the cause of any physical injuries. A perpetrator code (Y07) should be added when the perpetrator of the abuse is known. For suspected cases of abuse or neglect, do not report external cause or perpetrator code.	For use with any instance of abuse or neglect, in children or adults, perpetrator, or survivor. Also note the delineation between suspected and confirmed. These terms are best defined in a clinical policy for standardized utilization. Note: This guideline references the T-codes for abuse and neglect. There are other abuse and neglect codes, but they are located in the Y07 section of the Tabular Index.
V00–Y99 Codes	The external causes of morbidity codes should never be sequenced as the first-listed or principal diagnosis. They must accompany S- and T-codes and Injury and Poisoning codes must accompany External cause codes and Place of Occurrence codes as well. External cause codes are intended to provide data for injury research and evaluation of injury prevention strategies. These codes capture how the injury or health condition happened (cause), the intent (unintentional or accidental; or intentional, such as suicide or assault), the place where the event occurred, the activity of the patient at the time of the event, and the person's status (e.g., civilian, military). There is no national requirement for mandatory ICD-10-CM external cause code reporting. Unless a provider is	X71–X83: While "optional," this is a critical category for use in behavioral health regarding any suicide attempts. Tracking these X-codes, and seeing the possible progression of increasing lethality, may save a life. This is also important for national data and research on suicide and suicide prevention.

Item/ Condition	Coding and Documentation Guideline states:	Interpretation/ Comments
	subject to a state-based external cause code reporting mandate or these codes are required by a particular payer, reporting of ICD-10-CM codes in Chapter 20, External Causes of Morbidity, is not required. In the absence of a mandatory reporting requirement, providers are encouraged to voluntarily report external cause codes, as they provide valuable data for injury research and evaluation of injury prevention strategies.	
Child and Adult Abuse Guideline	Adult and child abuse, neglect and maltreatment are classified as assault. Any of the assault codes may be used to indicate the external cause of any injury resulting from the confirmed abuse. For confirmed cases of abuse, neglect and maltreatment, when the perpetrator is known, a code from Y07, Perpetrator of maltreatment and neglect, should accompany any other assault codes.	This is the Y07 section of the Tabular Index. Having a clinical policy, or training on these codes (compared to T-codes) will be essential for standardized utilization and data tracking purposes.
Use of Z-codes	Z-codes are for use in any healthcare setting. Z-codes may be used as either a first-listed (principal diagnosis code in the inpatient setting) or secondary code, depending on the circumstances of the encounter. Certain Z-codes may only be used as first-listed or principal diagnosis.	Z68 (BMI) category may be particularly useful for those who treat Eating Disorders; general screenings, counseling, psychosocial and socioeconomic factors impacting the clinical case are found here.
"History of" Z-codes	Personal history codes may be used in conjunction with follow-up codes and family history codes may be used in conjunction with screening codes to explain the need for a test or procedure. History codes are also acceptable on any medical record regardless of the reason for visit. A history of an illness, even if no longer present, is important information that may alter the type of treatment ordered. The history Z-code categories are: • Z81: Family history of mental and behavioral disorders	The utilization of these codes may be helpful to certain treatment settings or for research purposes. A clinical policy, or training, on the utilization of these codes is recommended for standardized utilization and data tracking purposes.

Table 2.4 *continued*

Item/ Condition	Coding and Documentation Guideline states:	Interpretation/ Comments
	• Z91.4-: Personal history of psychological trauma, not elsewhere classified • Z91.5: Personal history of self-harm	
Counseling Codes	Counseling Z-codes are used when a patient or family member receives assistance in the aftermath of an illness or injury, or when support is required in coping with family or social problems. • Z69: Encounter for mental health services for victim and perpetrator of abuse • Z70: Counseling related to sexual attitude, behavior and orientation	This may be of particular interest to those working in organizations that engage in the SAMSHA-HRSA "SBIRT" (Screening, Brief Intervention, and Referral to Treatment) integration program; also those working in medical settings may find these codes useful.
Miscellaneous Z-codes	The miscellaneous Z-codes capture a number of other healthcare encounters that do not fall into one of the other categories. Certain of these codes identify the reason for the encounter; others are for use as additional codes that provide useful information on circumstances that may affect a patient's care and treatment.	Self-explanatory
Inpatient Guidelines	The circumstances of inpatient admission always govern the selection of the principal diagnosis. The principal diagnosis is defined in the Uniform Hospital Discharge Data Set (UHDDS) as "that condition established after study to be chiefly responsible for occasioning the admission of the patient to the hospital for care." The UHDDS definitions are used by hospitals to report inpatient data elements in a standardized manner. These data elements and their definitions can be found in the July 31, 1985, Federal Register (Vol. 50, No, 147), pp. 31038–40. Since that time the application of the UHDDS definitions has been expanded	These inpatient guidelines will most likely apply to free-standing psychiatric hospitals, substance use facilities, and/or acute care facilities such as the psychiatric department of a general hospital.

Item/ Condition	Coding and Documentation Guideline states:	Interpretation/ Comments
	to include all non-outpatient settings (acute care, short-term, long-term care and psychiatric hospitals; home health agencies; rehab facilities; nursing homes, etc.). In determining principal diagnosis, coding conventions in the ICD-10-CM, the Tabular List and Alphabetic Index take precedence over these official coding guidelines. (See *Section I.A., Conventions for the ICD-10-CM.*) The importance of consistent, complete documentation in the medical record cannot be overemphasized. Without such documentation the application of all coding guidelines is a difficult, if not impossible, task.	
Uncertain Conditions (Inpatient)	If the diagnosis documented at the time of discharge is qualified as "probable," "suspected," "likely," "questionable," "possible," or "still to be ruled out," or other similar terms indicating uncertainty, code the condition as if it existed or was established. The bases for these guidelines are the diagnostic workup, arrangements for further workup or observation, and initial therapeutic approach that correspond most closely with the established diagnosis. Note: This guideline is applicable only to inpatient admissions to short-term, acute, long-term care and psychiatric hospitals.	Self-explanatory
Outpatient Guidelines	Coding guidelines for inconclusive diagnoses (probable, suspected, rule out, etc.) were developed for inpatient reporting and do not apply to outpatients. For accurate reporting of ICD-10-CM diagnosis codes, the documentation should describe the patient's condition, using terminology which includes specific diagnoses as well as symptoms, problems, or reasons for the encounter. There are ICD-10-CM codes to describe all of these.	This is a very clear, comprehensive guideline.

Table 2.4 *continued*

Item/ Condition	Coding and Documentation Guideline states:	Interpretation/ Comments
	ICD-10-CM is composed of codes with 3, 4, 5, 6 or 7 characters. Codes with 3 characters are included in ICD-10-CM as the heading of a category of codes that may be further subdivided by the use of fourth, fifth, sixth or seventh characters to provide greater specificity. A 3-character code is to be used only if it is not further subdivided. A code is invalid if it has not been coded to the full number of characters required for that code, including the 7th character, if applicable. Code all documented conditions that co-exist at the time of the encounter/ visit, and require or affect patient care treatment or management. Do not code conditions that were previously treated and no longer exist.	

Summary

In closing, there are several important issues to highlight from this chapter. They include the following:

1. Coding and documentation have historically been considered a medical industry standard of practice. Behavioral health clinicians are just as important as other providers in the healthcare industry. Having uniformity in our practices, documentation, and diagnostic labeling will facilitate quality consumer care and overall population health.
2. Behavioral health clinicians need to take ownership of where the diagnosis codes come from, and to where they are delivered. In other words, a clinician should not assume that the diagnosis assigned is the one that will appear on the claim form, or in data repositories.
3. Robust clinical documentation is important to facilitate comprehensive quality care and to demonstrate medical necessity. As HIPAA-covered entities, we are also mandated to follow the coding and documentation standards published by CMS and NCHS.
4. Two critical coding and documentation standards for behavioral health

clinicians are to diagnose to the highest level of specificity, and to be careful about our utilization of Unspecified and Other diagnoses. Behavioral health clinicians have a high incidence of assigning Unspecified or "NOS" diagnoses to their clients. Becoming specific will require a cultural shift, involving the obtaining of specific and detailed information from the client, and documenting to substantiate the assigned code number.

5. Several areas in coding and documentation require consideration of a standard policy and/or procedure to guide clinicians within an organization. For example, how medical diagnoses will get coded, and to what degree of specificity (i.e. how many characters in the ICD-10-CM), and this will need to be balanced according to the scope of practice laws and how best to provide your integrated care delivery model.

Bibliography

American Psychiatric Association. (2013). *Diagnostic and Statistical Manual of Mental Disorders: DSM-5* (pp. 15, 23, 491). Washington, DC: American Psychiatric Association.

Berwick, D. M., Nolan, T. W., & Whittington, J. (2008). The triple aim: Care, health, and cost. *Health Affairs, 27*(3), 759–69.

Blondeau, C., Ulbricht, M., & Dougherty, M. (Eds.). (2005). *Documentation and Reimbursement for Behavioral Health Services.* Chicago, IL: American Health Information Management Association.

Centers for Disease Control and Prevention. (2016). *International Classification of Diseases, Tenth Revision, Clinical Modification (ICD-10-CM), FY 2017 Guidelines*. Retrieved October 28, 2016 from www.cdc.gov/nchs/icd10cm.htm.

Centers for Medicare & Medicaid Services. (2016, March 11). *ICD-10.* Retrieved March 25, 2016 from www.cms.gov/medicare/Coding/ICD10/index.html.

Centers for Medicare & Medicaid Services. (2016, March 19). *ICD-10-CM Official Guidelines for Coding and Reporting FY 2016.* Retrieved March 25, 2016 from www.cms.gov/Medicare/Coding/ICD10/Downloads/2016-ICD-10-CM-Guidelines.pdf.

Office of Inspector General, Department of Health & Human Services. (1998). Publication of the OIG compliance program guidance for third-party medical billing companies. *Federal Register, 63*(243). Retrieved March 23, 2016 from http://oig.hhs.gov/fraud/docs/complianceguidance/thirdparty.pdf.

Social Security Administration. (n.d.). *Compilation of the Social Security Laws.* Retrieved March 25, 2016 from www.ssa.gov/OP_Home/ssact/title19/1902.htm.

3 Coding in the ICD Series: The Indices

This chapter will elaborate on the two indices used in the medical coding industry in the USA. Specifically, we will look at samples from the two indices pertaining to the delivery of behavioral health services and give explanations about their utilization. Keep in mind that the one, authoritative source for ICD series codes in the USA is the Tabular Index, which is found at the CDC's website in the ICD-10-CM section. Remember also that we are recommending that behavioral health clinicians utilize the Tabular Index even though the correct coding procedure is to use the Alphabetic Index first then the Tabular Index. We will spend the most time on the Tabular Index in this chapter.

Unlike the medical industry where Certified Professional Coders (CPCs) and/or encoders typically review medical record documentation for code accuracy, such checks and balances are not the norm in the behavioral health industry. As you will recall from previous discussions in this textbook, not all ICD-10-CM codes obtained from sources other than the Tabular Index are guaranteed clinically accurate. In fact, itemization of the ICD-10-CM codes from any source other than those endorsed by CMS can put providers at risk for revenue disruption and miscoding. However, there are an increasing number of behavioral health organizations that are employing CPCs to review charts, assign diagnoses, or even to verify diagnoses before they are submitted to a third party. It is anticipated that this practice will increase as regulatory compliance mandates continue to increase. Increased utilization of CPCs would benefit the behavioral health industry greatly.

The three main steps to assigning a diagnosis accurately in the medical industry can be:

1. Coder looks up the diagnostic term in the Alphabetic Index.
2. Coder looks up and verifies the code number in the Tabular Index.
3. Coder verifies that there are no specific reporting or coding guidelines that dictate the sequencing or utilization of the code chosen in #2 above.

More and more behavioral health clinicians may find themselves in a workplace that employs coders in some capacity. If the coders are CPCs, then it is important to understand that their thinking processes and tasks may differ greatly from those of the behavioral health clinician.

Coders will look at the clinical documentation in the medical record and assign the most specific diagnosis to the condition treated during that healthcare encounter, unless they use an encoder. Clinicians, on the other hand, will assign the diagnosis according to criteria outlined in the ICD or DSM, and the corresponding diagnosis code should have sufficient documentation in the record to substantiate the diagnosis assigned. Both coders and clinicians will use the Tabular Index and perhaps the Alphabetic Index as well, depending on the circumstances.

The Alphabetic Index

The Alphabetic Index in the ICD-10-CM consists of an alphabetic index formatted by main terms listed in alphabetic order, with indentations for any applicable qualifiers or descriptors. It is an alphabetical list of terms used to describe disease conditions, by specific illness, abbreviation, injury, or other descriptive diagnostic term. Terms used for other reasons for the healthcare encounter are also listed in the Alphabetic Index.

The process for using the Alphabetic Index is to look up the main term written in the medical record in the Index, scan the sub terms as appropriate, then move into the Tabular Index to locate the most accurate diagnostic code. For example, a psychiatrist may write in the medical record "Asocial personality" and not assign a diagnosis code. The coder, in turn, must determine what diagnosis code number to assign to the episode of care:

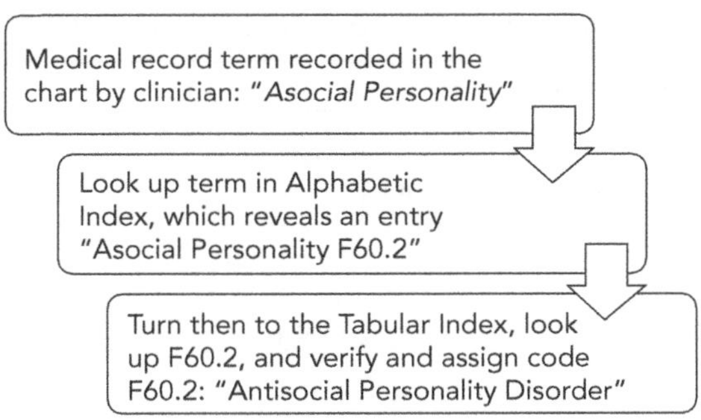

While a clinician is not likely to go through this process, administrators, billing office personnel, internal auditing committees and compliance may find this information useful. Justifying the assigned diagnosis code with the medical record documentation, or submitted code to the third-party payer, is critically important for program integrity audits performed by the Office of the Inspector General (OIG). The OIG is in charge of mitigating fraud, waste, and abuse, and they often do this, in part, by reviewing the clinical documentation of the submitted, or claimed, diagnosis.

Alphabetic Index Samples:

Table 3.1 Asocial Personality Disorder, Alphabetic Index, page 119

2016 Alphabetic Index
Askin's tumor – see Neoplasm, connective tissue, malignant
Asocial personality F60.2
Asomatognosia R41.4
Aspartylglucosaminuria E77.1
Asperger's disease or syndrome F84.5
Aspergilloma – see Aspergillosis

You will note in Table 3.1 above that "Asocial personality" is listed in alphabetical order amid all the other diagnostic, medical terms. Keep in mind the Alphabetic Index is over 1,300 pages long so it contains a tremendous volume of terms and diagnoses. Coders will use this Index to help them find the right section in the Tabular Index to assign the correct code. In this example, the Alphabetic Index is suggesting that the coder look at F60.2 in the Tabular Index for the correct diagnosis code. Another good example of commingled health conditions is in the Depression section. We listed just a few here as examples in Table 3.2:

Table 3.2 Depression Section, Alphabetic Index, pages 360–1

Depression (acute) (mental) F32.9
agitated (single episode) F32.2
anaclitic – *see* Disorder, adjustment
anxiety F41.8
persistent F34.1
arches – *see also* Deformity, limb, flat foot

atypical (single episode) F32.8
basal metabolic rate R94.8
bone marrow D75.89

Other samples from the Depression section
hysterical F44.89
major F32.9
with psychotic symptoms F32.3
recurrent – *see* Disorder, depressive, recurrent
neurotic F34.1
postpartum F53
psychoneurotic F34.1
seasonal – *see* Disorder, depressive, recurrent
skull Q67.4

The Tabular Index

While those in the certified coding Industry across all disciplines in healthcare typically follow the process of Alphabetic Index to Tabular Index, encouraging behavioral health clinicians to utilize the specificity of the index has proved challenging. This distinction begs the question: "Why is the Tabular Index so important? Why should behavioral health professionals bother with this Index when they have other means of accessing ICD-10-CM codes for diagnosing and reimbursement purposes?" The answer is straightforward and simple: if you are a HIPAA-covered entity, you are required to use the ICD-10-CM codes to be in full compliance with the regulations. CMS, in the Frequently Asked Questions (FAQ) section, number 1817, further indicates that code assignments originate from the following sources:

- ICD-10-CM Code Books
- Specialty Specific Code Books
- Electronic versions of ICD-10-CM found on the CMS and CDC website
- Encoders.

The FAQ goes on to indicate that while there are ICD-10-CM code values notated in the DSM-5 book, those codes were assigned by the APA. The NCHS and CDC revise the Tabular Index twice a year, and it is the one resource utilized by all healthcare stakeholders, including the third-party payers in the USA. The most recent itemization of the ICD can be found on the CDC website, and it is downloadable for easy access.

As we know, there are 21 Chapters in the Tabular Index. Behavioral health clinicians will want to familiarize themselves not only with Chapter 5, but also with every other chapter and family of codes that pertain to their client population (see Table 3.3). The remainder of this chapter will take an in-depth look at the Tabular Index coding system, with explanations about utilization.

Table 3.3 The 2017 ICD-10-CM Tabular Index Table of Contents

The 2017 ICD-10-CM Tabular List of Diseases and Injuries		
Chapter	**Category/Condition**	**Code Block Number**
1	Certain infectious and parasitic diseases	A00–B99
2	Neoplasms	C00–D49
3	Diseases of the blood and blood-forming organs and certain disorders involving the immune mechanism	D50–D89
4	Endocrine, nutritional and metabolic diseases	E00–E89
5	Mental, behavioral and neurodevelopmental disorders	F01–F99
6	Diseases of the nervous system	G00–G99
7	Diseases of the eye and adnexa	H00–H59
8	Diseases of the ear and mastoid process	H60–H95
9	Diseases of the circulatory system	I00–I99
10	Diseases of the respiratory system	J00–J99
11	Diseases of the digestive system	K00-K95
12	Diseases of the skin and subcutaneous tissue	L00–L99
13	Diseases of the musculoskeletal system and connective tissue	M00–M99
14	Diseases of the genitourinary system	N00–N99
15	Pregnancy, childbirth and the puerperium	O00–O9A
16	Certain conditions originating in the perinatal period	P00–P96
17	Congenital malformations, deformations and chromosomal abnormalities	Q00–Q99
18	Symptoms, signs and abnormal clinical and laboratory findings, not elsewhere classified	R00–R99
19	Injury, poisoning and certain other consequences of external causes	S00–T88
20	External causes of morbidity	V00–Y99
21	Factors influencing health status and contact with health services	Z00–Z99

Mental Health Codes

For most behavioral health entities, codes from Chapters 5 and 21 will be the most frequently used. These F- and Z-codes are easily displayed in a tiered format, in numerical order. Keep in mind the coding and documentation guidelines from Chapter 2 tell us to use the most specific ICD-10-CM code possible. When looking at the Tabular Index, the level of specificity is very easy to visually identify. However, in many EHR systems where the codes are itemized or listed in a single drop-down box, it may be more difficult to discern which codes in a grouping are actually the most specific ones available.

The first few pages of the Tabular Index provide the Table of Contents and "Instructional Notations"; these notations are the coding and documentation guidelines put into practice in the Tabular Index. We will now look at select groupings of diagnoses in the 2017 Tabular Index and discuss the interpretation of the actual codes.

Major Depression, Single Episode

F32 Major depressive disorder, single episode
Includes: single episode of agitated depression
single episode of depressive reaction
single episode of major depression
single episode of psychogenic depression
single episode of reactive depression
single episode of vital depression
Excludes1: bipolar disorder (F31.-)
manic episode (F30.-)
recurrent depressive disorder (F33.-)
Excludes2: adjustment disorder (F43.2)

F32.0 Major depressive disorder, single episode, mild

F32.1 Major depressive disorder, single episode, moderate

F32.2 Major depressive disorder, single episode, severe without psychotic features

F32.3 Major depressive disorder, single episode, severe with psychotic features
Single episode of major depression with mood-congruent psychotic symptoms
Single episode of major depression with mood-incongruent psychotic symptoms

Single episode of major depression with psychotic symptoms
Single episode of psychogenic depressive psychosis
Single episode of psychotic depression
Single episode of reactive depressive psychosis

F32.4 Major depressive disorder, single episode, in partial remission

F32.5 Major depressive disorder, single episode, in full remission

F32.8 Other depressive episodes

F32.81 Premenstrual dysphoric disorder
Excludes1: premenstrual tension syndrome (N94.3)

F32.89 Other specified depressive episodes
Atypical depression
Post-schizophrenic depression
Single episode of "masked" depression NOS

F32.9 Major depressive disorder, single episode, unspecified
Depression NOS
Depressive disorder NOS
Major depression NOS

Author's Interpretation Notes:

Bolded Items: The names of diagnoses and/or instructions on how to use a category or diagnosis.

Plain Text: 1. An alternative way of describing the condition, perhaps language used in medical chart notes by a clinician. 2. Plain text may also indicate the name that the APA or US has given to the condition, and this may/may not be recognized internationally. Sometimes the APA or US has a unique diagnosis in bold in the ICD-10-CM and it may not be recognized in other ICD-10 classifications. 3. Also, plain text may represent other possible diagnoses in the section that are to be included in the Bolded coding number above it.

In looking at the example above, we can extract and determine the following about Major Depression, Single Episode:

- F32 is considered a 3-character code because it takes up three digit spaces, and is called a *category* heading.
- F32.1 is a 4-character code.

- 4-character codes are the most specific diagnoses available in this category since there are no 5-, 6-, or 7-character codes listed in this category.
- The word "includes" under some diagnoses or categories further defines the diagnosis, or gives examples of presenting conditions of the client that should be considered in that particular category.
- "Excludes1" indicates that you should NOT diagnose those particular conditions at the same time as you assign the Category heading diagnosis. In other words, do not diagnose Manic episode at the same time as you assign the diagnosis of Major Depression, Single Episode. Instead, the Tabular Index refers you to the F30 category for the Mania diagnoses.
- "Excludes2" indicates that you CAN diagnose these conditions simultaneously. For example, you CAN diagnose a Single Episode of Major Depression concurrent with an Adjustment Disorder.
- If you have a client with "Atypical Depression," then you are to assign F32.8, "Other Depressive Episodes" to the healthcare encounter.
- If you have a client with "Depression NOS," then you assign F32.9, Major Depressive Disorder, Single Episode, Unspecified.

There are some other considerations when choosing a diagnosis, especially in the US healthcare industry:

1. While F32 is a diagnosis, many third-party payers will require a reportable code. F32 is not reportable because it is a category heading and further subdivided.
2. Some third-party entities may "claim edit" or "claim review" 3-character codes as not reportable. Claim edits are computer programs to identify any codes that may not be legitimate or deemed sufficient. This may result in delayed reimbursements, or outright claim denials that may need to be appealed. This could be problematic because there are several 3-character codes that are not further subdivided in Chapter 5 (e.g. F70: Mild intellectual disabilities; F53: Puerperal Psychosis).
3. NOS, Unspecified, or Other diagnoses tend to be over-utilized in the behavioral health industry. It is not uncommon for an organization to pull a report of their "Top 10" diagnoses and find a large portion of those be unspecified. There are benefits as well as challenges to this practice, which will be discussed in Chapter 6.

When documenting to support the diagnosis, it is incumbent upon the clinician to account for every element in the assigned code or diagnosis in the client chart. One suggestion for accomplishing this objective is to document each critical word found in the diagnosis name or label. For example, let us look at F32.3, Major Depressive Disorder, Single Episode, Severe With Psychotic Features:

- What are the diagnostic criteria used to reach this conclusion?
- Where did you get the diagnostic criteria for making the diagnosis?
- Are the diagnostic criteria itemized in the record to support this diagnosis?
- Why is this a Single Episode versus a Recurrent Episode?
- How do you account for the severity rating of Severe?
- What are the Psychotic Features or symptoms that warrant this particular diagnosis?

Post-Traumatic Stress Disorder (PTSD)

F43 Reaction to severe stress, and adjustment disorders

F43.0 Acute stress reaction
Acute crisis reaction
Acute reaction to stress
Combat and operational stress reaction
Combat fatigue
Crisis state
Psychic shock

F43.1 Post-traumatic stress disorder (PTSD)
Traumatic neurosis

F43.10 Post-traumatic stress disorder, unspecified

F43.11 Post-traumatic stress disorder, acute

F43.12 Post-traumatic stress disorder, chronic

In assessing the options in the PTSD category, we can interpret the available information in the following manner:

- There are three subdivisions to PTSD: unspecified, acute, and chronic.
- F43.1 will likely not be an acceptable diagnosis for purposes of reimbursement by third parties in the USA because there are subdivisions available.

Note: the DSM-5 only gives us one code for PTSD: *F43.10 Post-Traumatic Stress Disorder, Unspecified*. While the DSM-5 does indicate to choose a written specifier for acute versus chronic states, there is no assigned code or digit used to reflect the acute versus chronic status, as is done in the ICD-10-CM. This absence can be problematic for a variety of reasons:

- Third-party payers may not (and have not in some cases) accept the unspecified diagnosis, either in the short term or long term.
- Specifiers written in the text portion of the medical record are not easily accessible.
- Unless the PTSD-Acute or Chronic codes are easily accessible, concurrent or subsequent, clinicians will have to read through the medical record to figure out if this is an acute or chronic condition.
- The diagnostic criteria for distinguishing between acute versus chronic are not delineated in either the DSM-5 or the ICD-10 CDDG.

Eating Disorders

F50 Eating disorders
Excludes1: anorexia NOS (R63.0)
feeding difficulties (R63.3)
polyphagia (R63.2)
Excludes2: feeding disorder in infancy or childhood (F98.2-)
F50.0 Anorexia nervosa
Excludes1: loss of appetite (R63.0)
psychogenic loss of appetite (F50.8)
F50.00 Anorexia nervosa, unspecified
F50.01 Anorexia nervosa, restricting type
F50.02 Anorexia nervosa, binge-eating/purging type
Excludes1: bulimia nervosa (F50.2)
F50.2 Bulimia nervosa
Bulimia NOS
Hyperorexia nervosa
Excludes1: anorexia nervosa, binge-eating/purging type (F50.02)
F50.8 Other eating disorders
Excludes2: pica of infancy and childhood (F98.3)
F50.81 Binge-Eating Disorder
F50.89 Other specified eating disorder
Pica in adults
Psychogenic loss of appetite
F50.9 Eating disorder, unspecified
Atypical anorexia nervosa
Atypical bulimia nervosa

The Eating Disorders category in the Tabular Index is straightforward in its delineation of diagnoses. However, as will be discussed in Chapter 4, there are some challenges to deciding how to code some of the eating disorders from the DSM-5. For example, F50.8 in the DSM-5 has been assigned to three different diagnoses: Avoidant/restrictive food intake disorder, Other specified feeding or eating disorder, and Pica in adults. Looking at the code number alone, it will be uncertain which diagnosis was actually intended unless the text narrative portion of the medical record is reviewed.

Keep in mind that CMS and third-party payers keep "profiling metrics" on clinicians as a means to track quality of care. Over-utilization of Other or Unspecified diagnoses can put the clinician at higher risk for audits, but in some cases such diagnoses will be unavoidable. To cope with this challenge, it is best to have a clinical policy and procedure in place that outline the circumstances in which an Other or Unspecified diagnosis is warranted.

In looking at the Eating Disorders in the Tabular Index, we see several instances of Excludes1 or Excludes2. Some of the sections in the Tabular Index have more instructional notations than others. Some comments on this category include:

- F50.0 is a category heading for Anorexia Nervosa.
- Anorexia Nervosa has three subdivisions, or different types to choose from and they are 5-character codes.
- Since F50.0 is not as specific as the 5-character codes, the more-specific 5-character code will likely be mandated or required by third-party stakeholders.

Intellectual Disabilities

Intellectual Disabilities (F70–F79)
Code First any associated physical or developmental disorders
Excludes1: borderline intellectual functioning, IQ above 70 to 84 (R41.83)

F70 Mild intellectual disabilities
IQ level 50–55 to approximately 70
Mild mental subnormality

F71 Moderate intellectual disabilities
IQ level 35–40 to 50–55
Moderate mental subnormality

F72 Severe intellectual disabilities
IQ 20–25 to 35–40
Severe mental subnormality

F73 Profound intellectual disabilities
IQ level below 20–25
Profound mental subnormality

F78 Other intellectual disabilities

F79 Unspecified intellectual disabilities
Mental deficiency NOS
Mental subnormality NOS

The Intellectual Disabilities is an interesting section in the Tabular Index for a variety of reasons. First, each diagnosis is only at the 3-character code level and there are no further subdivisions. Next, it appears that to assign these diagnoses, a clinician would need to know the Intelligence Quotient (IQ) numerical levels of the client in order to assign the severity levels. One option if the IQ levels are not known is to use the Unspecified category until the IQ levels can be obtained and documented. However, long-term use of an Unspecified diagnosis may be problematic in this population for a variety of stakeholders.

The most interesting part of this section is the Instructional Notations of "Code First" and "Excludes1". There is an implication with the "Code First" rule that physical health conditions are documented and assigned first when listing multiple diagnoses. Keep in mind that this can present problems for some in the behavioral health industry, for example:

- Some professionals who might be practicing outside their scope of competence or licensure by assigning a medical diagnosis.
- Some third-party entities, such as payers for reimbursement, who may only reimburse for these codes if the facility or clinician is a designated treatment provider for individuals with these conditions.

The "Excludes1" notation directs cases in which the IQ is above 70–84 to assign a code from another Chapter in the Tabular Index altogether, Chapter 18's Symptoms, Signs and Abnormal Clinical and Laboratory Findings, Not Elsewhere Classified (i.e. the R-codes). This situation is an excellent example of why behavioral health clinicians will need access to the *entire* Tabular Index, not just Chapter 5's Mental and Behavioral and Neurodevelopmental Disorders.

The clinician's job is to assign the most accurate and specific diagnosis applicable for any healthcare encounter. Most payers have an itemization of covered versus not-covered diagnoses; not all codes, however, are going to be "reimbursable" by third-party payers in the USA. The terminology used for this typically is "billable" versus "not-billable."

Disorders with Onset in Childhood and Adolescence

F91 Conduct disorders
Excludes1: antisocial behavior (Z72.81-)
antisocial personality disorder (F60.2)
Excludes2: conduct problems associated with attention-deficit hyperactivity disorder (F90.-)
mood [affective] disorders (F30-F39)
pervasive developmental disorders (F84.-)
schizophrenia (F20.-)

F91.0 Conduct disorder confined to family context

F91.1 Conduct disorder, childhood-onset type
Unsocialized conduct disorder
Conduct disorder, solitary aggressive type
Unsocialized aggressive disorder

F91.2 Conduct disorder, adolescent-onset type
Socialized conduct disorder
Conduct disorder, group type

F91.3 Oppositional defiant disorder

F91.8 Other conduct disorders
Other specified conduct disorder
Other specified disruptive disorder NOS

F91.9 Conduct disorder, unspecified
Behavioral disorder NOS
Conduct disorder NOS
Disruptive behavior disorder NOS
Disruptive disorder NOS

As discussed in Chapter 4, there are some differences between the ICD-10-CM Childhood category and how the child and adolescent disorders are incorporated throughout the entire DSM-5. Having these disorders grouped together is actually helpful when choosing a diagnosis grouping. It is important to point out that F91.0 Conduct Disorder Confined to Family Context is a diagnosis exclusive to the ICD-10-CM at the time of this writing. This particular diagnosis can be beneficial to certain populations and facilities.

Psychoactive Substance Use Disorders

F10.9 Alcohol use, unspecified
Excludes1: alcohol abuse (F10.1-)
alcohol dependence (F10.2-)

F10.92 Alcohol use, unspecified with intoxication
F10.920 Alcohol use, unspecified with intoxication, uncomplicated
F10.921 Alcohol use, unspecified with intoxication delirium
F10.929 Alcohol use, unspecified with intoxication, unspecified

F10.94 Alcohol use, unspecified with alcohol-induced mood disorder use
Alcohol-induced bipolar or related disorder, without use disorder
Alcohol-induced depressive disorder, without use disorder

F10.95 Alcohol use, unspecified with alcohol-induced psychotic disorder
F10.950 Alcohol use, unspecified with alcohol-induced psychotic disorder with delusions
F10.951 Alcohol use, unspecified with alcohol-induced psychotic disorder with hallucinations
F10.959 Alcohol use, unspecified with alcohol-induced psychotic disorder, unspecified
Alcohol-induced psychotic disorder without use disorder

F10.96 Alcohol use, unspecified with alcohol-induced persisting amnestic disorder
Alcohol-induced major neurocognitive disorder, amnestic-confabulatory type, without use disorder

F10.97 Alcohol use, unspecified with alcohol-induced persisting dementia
Alcohol-induced major neurocognitive disorder, nonamnestic-confabulatory type, without use disorder

F10.98 Alcohol use, unspecified with other alcohol-induced disorders

F10.980 Alcohol use, unspecified with alcohol-induced anxiety disorder
Alcohol-induced anxiety disorder, without use disorder

F10.981 Alcohol use, unspecified with alcohol-induced sexual dysfunction
Alcohol-induced sexual dysfunction, without use disorder

F10.982 Alcohol use, unspecified with alcohol-induced sleep disorder
Alcohol-induced sleep disorder, without use disorder

F10.988 Alcohol use, unspecified with other alcohol-induced disorder
Alcohol-induced mild neurocognitive disorder, without use disorder

F10.99 Alcohol use, unspecified with unspecified alcohol-induced disorder

F12 Cannabis related disorders
Includes: marijuana

F12.1 Cannabis abuse
Excludes1: cannabis dependence (F12.2-)
cannabis use, unspecified (F12.9-)

F12.10 Cannabis abuse, uncomplicated
Cannabis use disorder, mild

F12.12 Cannabis abuse with intoxication
F12.120 Cannabis abuse with intoxication, uncomplicated
F12.121 Cannabis abuse with intoxication delirium
F12.122 Cannabis abuse with intoxication with perceptual disturbance
F12.129 Cannabis abuse with intoxication, unspecified

F12.15 Cannabis abuse with psychotic disorder
F12.150 Cannabis abuse with psychotic disorder with delusions
F12.151 Cannabis abuse with psychotic disorder with hallucinations

F12.159 Cannabis abuse with psychotic disorder, unspecified

F12.18 Cannabis abuse with other cannabis-induced disorder

F12.180 Cannabis abuse with cannabis-induced anxiety disorder

F12.188 Cannabis abuse with other cannabis-induced disorder

Cannabis use disorder, mild, with cannabis-induced sleep disorder

F12.19 Cannabis abuse with unspecified cannabis-induced disorder

F13.2 Sedative, hypnotic or anxiolytic-related dependence

Excludes1: sedative, hypnotic or anxiolytic-related abuse (F13.1-)
sedative, hypnotic, or anxiolytic use, unspecified (F13.9-)

Excludes2: sedative, hypnotic, or anxiolytic poisoning (T42.-)

F13.20 Sedative, hypnotic or anxiolytic dependence, uncomplicated

F13.21 Sedative, hypnotic or anxiolytic dependence, in remission

F13.22 Sedative, hypnotic or anxiolytic dependence with intoxication

Excludes1: sedative, hypnotic or anxiolytic dependence with withdrawal (F13.23-)

F13.220 Sedative, hypnotic or anxiolytic dependence with intoxication, uncomplicated

F13.221 Sedative, hypnotic or anxiolytic dependence with intoxication delirium

F13.229 Sedative, hypnotic or anxiolytic dependence with intoxication, unspecified

F13.23 Sedative, hypnotic or anxiolytic dependence with withdrawal

Sedative, hypnotic, or anxiolytic use disorder, moderate
Sedative, hypnotic, or anxiolytic use disorder, severe

Excludes1: sedative, hypnotic or anxiolytic dependence with intoxication (F13.22-)

F13.230 Sedative, hypnotic or anxiolytic dependence with withdrawal, uncomplicated

F13.231 Sedative, hypnotic or anxiolytic dependence with withdrawal delirium

F13.232 Sedative, hypnotic or anxiolytic dependence with withdrawal with perceptual disturbance

F13.239 Sedative, hypnotic or anxiolytic dependence with withdrawal, unspecified

Sedative, hypnotic, or anxiolytic withdrawal with perceptual disturbances

F13.24 Sedative, hypnotic or anxiolytic dependence with sedative, hypnotic or anxiolytic-induced mood disorder

Sedative, hypnotic or anxiolytic use disorder, moderate, with sedative, hypnotic or anxiolytic-induced bipolar or related disorder

Sedative, hypnotic or anxiolytic use disorder, moderate, hypnotic or anxiolytic-induced depressive disorder

Sedative, hypnotic or anxiolytic use disorder, severe, with sedative, hypnotic or anxiolytic-induced bipolar or related disorder

Sedative, hypnotic or anxiolytic use disorder, severe, hypnotic or anxiolytic-induced depressive disorder

F13.25 Sedative, hypnotic or anxiolytic dependence with sedative, hypnotic or anxiolytic-induced psychotic disorder

F13.250 Sedative, hypnotic or anxiolytic dependence with sedative, hypnotic or anxiolytic- induced psychotic disorder with delusions

F13.251 Sedative, hypnotic or anxiolytic dependence with sedative, hypnotic or anxiolytic- induced psychotic disorder with hallucinations

F13.259 Sedative, hypnotic or anxiolytic dependence with sedative, hypnotic or anxiolytic- induced psychotic disorder, unspecified

F13.26 Sedative, hypnotic or anxiolytic dependence with sedative, hypnotic or anxiolytic-induced persisting amnestic disorder

F13.27 Sedative, hypnotic or anxiolytic dependence with sedative, hypnotic or anxiolytic-induced persisting dementia

Sedative, hypnotic or anxiolytic use disorder, moderate, with sedative, hypnotic or anxiolytic-induced major neurocognitive disorder

Sedative, hypnotic or anxiolytic use disorder, severe, with sedative, hypnotic or anxiolytic-induced major neurocognitive disorder

F13.28 Sedative, hypnotic or anxiolytic dependence with other sedative, hypnotic or anxiolytic-induced disorders

F13.280 Sedative, hypnotic or anxiolytic dependence with sedative, hypnotic or anxiolytic-induced anxiety disorder

F13.281 Sedative, hypnotic or anxiolytic dependence with sedative, hypnotic or anxiolytic- induced sexual dysfunction

F13.282 Sedative, hypnotic or anxiolytic dependence with sedative, hypnotic or anxiolytic-induced sleep disorder

F13.288 Sedative, hypnotic or anxiolytic dependence with other sedative, hypnotic or anxiolytic-induced disorder

Sedative, hypnotic or anxiolytic use disorder, moderate, with sedative, hypnotic or anxiolytic-induced major neurocognitive disorder

Sedative, hypnotic or anxiolytic use disorder, severe, with sedative, hypnotic or anxiolytic-induced major neurocognitive disorder

F13.29 Sedative, hypnotic or anxiolytic dependence with unspecified sedative, hypnotic or anxiolytic-induced disorder

F17 Nicotine dependence

Excludes1: history of tobacco dependence (Z87.891)
tobacco use NOS (Z72.0)

Excludes2: tobacco use (smoking) during pregnancy, childbirth and the puerperium (O99.33-)
toxic effect of nicotine (T65.2-)

F17.2 Nicotine dependence

F17.20 Nicotine dependence, unspecified

F17.200 Nicotine dependence, unspecified, uncomplicated
Tobacco use disorder, mild
Tobacco use disorder, moderate
Tobacco use disorder, severe

F17.201 Nicotine dependence, unspecified, in remission

F17.203 Nicotine dependence unspecified, with withdrawal
Tobacco withdrawal

F17.208 Nicotine dependence, unspecified, with other nicotine-induced disorders

F17.209 Nicotine dependence, unspecified, with unspecified nicotine-induced disorders

F17.21 Nicotine dependence, cigarettes

F17.210 Nicotine dependence, cigarettes, uncomplicated

F17.211 Nicotine dependence, cigarettes, in remission

F17.213 Nicotine dependence, cigarettes, with withdrawal

F17.218 Nicotine dependence, cigarettes, with other nicotine-induced disorders

F17.219 Nicotine dependence, cigarettes, with unspecified nicotine-induced disorders

F17.22 Nicotine dependence, chewing tobacco

F17.220 Nicotine dependence, chewing tobacco, uncomplicated

F17.221 Nicotine dependence, chewing tobacco, in remission

F17.223 Nicotine dependence, chewing tobacco, with withdrawal

F17.228 Nicotine dependence, chewing tobacco, with other nicotine-induced disorders

F17.229 **Nicotine dependence, chewing tobacco, with unspecified nicotine-induced disorders**

F17.29 **Nicotine dependence, other tobacco product**

F17.290 **Nicotine dependence, other tobacco product, uncomplicated**

F17.291 **Nicotine dependence, other tobacco product, in remission**

F17.293 **Nicotine dependence, other tobacco product, with withdrawal**

F17.298 **Nicotine dependence, other tobacco product, with other nicotine-induced disorders**

F17.299 **Nicotine dependence, other tobacco product, with unspecified nicotine-induced disorders**

The psychoactive substance use category is quite extensive in the Tabular Index. It is especially helpful to look at this chapter on paper, or in PDF format downloaded from the CDC website. The delineations, subcategories, and the sheer number of available diagnoses are extensive. To give you a sense of the Substance Use Diagnoses in the Tabular Index, several sections are displayed in this text: 1. Alcohol Use, 2. Cannabis Related Disorders, 3. Sedative, Hypnotic or Anxiolytic Dependence, and 4. Nicotine Dependence.

If you recall, the ICD-10-CM differs from the DSM-5 in that the categorizations for Substance Use retain the "Use, Abuse, and Dependence" structure whereas the DSM-5 uses the categories of "Use or Induced" to reflect a more dimensional approach. Also, because of the expansive nature of this set of diagnoses, the documentation requirements or elements are going to be significantly more than for some of the other diagnoses in Chapter 5.

Finally, it is critical to point out that there are instances of two different disorders being assigned the same code number in the DSM-5, with a trickle-down effect into the ICD-10-CM which is confusing for everyone. A concrete example of this is the code number F10.20:

- F10.20 in the Tabular Index is Alcohol dependence, uncomplicated;
- F10.20 in the DSM-5 is Alcohol use disorder, moderate;
- F10.20 in the DSM-5 is Alcohol use disorder, severe.

The lack of differentiation in the code numbers for differing diagnoses is problematic for everyone, and especially for accurate documentation and representation of the client's condition. The distinction between moderate and severe can also make a difference in treatment planning and levels of care provided. In other words, the code number in this instance is problematic because it is not clear what is the true diagnosis.

Class Discussion

Substance Use in the Tabular Index

From the samples above, discuss:

- What patterns do you notice across the substances?
- Are there some diagnoses that do not seem that much different from another, and yet they are assigned two different code values? What is the difference? How would this be interpreted by different clinicians?
- To support the ICD-10-CM diagnoses of Substance Use, Abuse, and Dependence, where would you get the clinical criteria and what would you have to document in the medical record? (Hint: the criteria are not listed in the DSM-5!)
- How likely is it that you will be able to memorize the code numbers?

If these diagnoses are itemized in a drop-down menu, how easy might it be to accidentally choose the wrong diagnosis because you lifted your finger off the mouse just one nanosecond too soon?

Physical Health Codes and Suicide Attempt/ Intentional Self-Harm Codes

This section of Chapter 3 will take you through some of the physical health or related codes that are useful to behavioral health clinicians when providing a comprehensive diagnosis of a client. The Affordable Care Act calls for better healthcare service delivery to those with co-morbid behavioral and physical health conditions. Part of the newer service delivery models include the concept called "Integrated Behavioral Health," and the Agency for Healthcare Research and Quality (AHRQ) defines this as:

> The care a patient experiences as a result of a team of primary care and behavioral health clinicians, working together with patients and families, using a systematic and cost-effective approach to provide patient-centered care for a defined population.
>
> (Agency for Healthcare Research and Quality, n.d.)

In March 2014, President Obama signed the Protecting Access to Medicare Act of 2014. In this legislation, there were provisions for the Excellence in Mental Health Act to help design and develop groundbreaking behavioral health service delivery models across the USA. Specifically, Section 223, Demonstration Program for Certified Community Behavioral Health Clinics, gives the details of this program. The legislation gave states the opportunity to participate in a demonstration project involving the Certified Community Behavioral Health Center (CCBHC), which is a national initiative to standardize and improve the delivery of behavioral health care services. Even if an organization or state is choosing not to participate in this exciting initiative, CCBHCs are likely to be the new gold standard in the industry for providing quality, comprehensive, whole-person care moving into the future.

There are many regulatory requirements that both organizations and states must meet to participate in the CCBHC initiatives. Among the many requirements is the ability for both organizations and states to meet minimum standards in several areas, one notably in quality reporting. Like other CMS Quality Reporting Initiatives such as the Physician's Quality Reporting System (PQRS), participating entities must track and report a number of quality measures in order to meet the minimum participation standards. At the time of this writing, states must send back to the federal government a number of quality metrics. One of those measures is "Number of Suicide Deaths and/or Attempts Requiring Medical Services by Patients Engaged in Behavioral Health (CCBHC) Treatment."

In addition to reporting metrics on suicide deaths and/or attempts, other metrics and requirements that the Substance Abuse and Mental Health Services Administration (SAMHSA) Planning Grants state that must be met are:

- assessments of suicide risk
- cultural competency training regarding suicide prevention
- identification of suicide risk factors.

These are critical points to take into consideration because it becomes evident that these items must be tracked either by claims data reviews or via reporting in the EHR as standardized data elements. What could this mean? It means that clinicians will need to utilize the entire ICD-10-CM X-code section, Intentional Self-Harm, to meet these reporting requirements in the future.

What are the most common co-morbid physical health conditions in the behavioral health population? More importantly, how do we as behavioral healthcare clinicians document, diagnose, and code for physical health and self-harm conditions? Keep in mind that if you just put a notation of the physical health or self-harm condition in the *narrative portion of the medical record*, it may not populate on the cover or face sheet, be traceable as reportable data, be analyzed in claims data reviews, or be included in the list of diagnoses being addressed, and therefore potentially go unnoticed by care providers.

We will look at the following three physical health conditions in the Tabular Index: Diabetes, Hypertension, and Obesity. The samples below have been streamlined from the way they are laid out in the Tabular Index for demonstration purposes. The main rationale for this is that as behavioral health clinicians, we will not be giving highly specific physical health diagnoses to the populations we serve. The degree of specificity assigned will need to be an internal discussion, and ideally a Clinical Policy and Procedure will be developed to help guide clinicians when diagnosing physical health issues. Again, it would be useful to look at these sections directly in the Tabular Index.

Diabetes mellitus (E08-E13)

E10 Type 1 diabetes mellitus

E10.3 Type 1 diabetes mellitus with opthalmic complications

E10.31 Type 1 diabetes mellitus with unspecified diabetic retinopathy

E10.311 Type 1 diabetes mellitus with unspecified diabetic retinopathy with macular edema

E10.319 Type 1 diabetes mellitus with unspecified diabetic retinopathy without macular edema

Hypertension Section

I13 Hypertensive heart and chronic kidney disease

I13.0 Hypertensive heart and chronic kidney disease with heart failure and stage 1 through stage 4 chronic kidney disease, or unspecified chronic kidney disease

I13.1 Hypertensive heart and chronic kidney disease without heart failure

I13.10 Hypertensive heart and chronic kidney disease without heart failure, with stage 1 through stage 4 chronic kidney disease, or unspecified chronic kidney disease

I13.11 Hypertensive heart and chronic kidney disease without heart failure, with stage 5 chronic kidney disease, or end stage renal disease

Overweight, obesity and other hyperalimentation (E65-E68)

E65 Localized adiposity

E66 Overweight and obesity

E66.0 Obesity due to excess calories

E66.01 Morbid (severe) obesity due to excess calories

E66.09 Other obesity due to excess calories

E66.1 Drug-induced obesity

E66.2 Morbid (severe) obesity with alveolar hypoventilation

Pickwickian syndrome

E66.3 Overweight

E66.8 Other obesity

E66.9 Obesity, unspecified Obesity NOS

Class Discussion:

Considerations for Medical Coding/Diagnosing

- The Tabular Index makes the subdivisions in the medical diagnostic sections clear. To what degree are you comfortable assigning a code number? A 3-character code? 4-5-6-characters?
- What are the implications if you do not assign a code number to a case where the individual is both seriously mentally ill AND who has some of the serious co-morbid conditions such as obesity or hypertension?
- How will you track suicide attempts as structured data? Are the X-codes sufficient?
- What is your role as the behavioral health clinician in helping keep track of your client's medical issues? Is your agency's reimbursement by third-party payers contingent on tracking and monitoring for physical health improvements?
- Does your practice setting make a difference in how you might assign codes, e.g. you work in a Patient-Centered Medical Home, Integrated Care setting, private practice with psychotherapy only, versus a community behavioral health center (i.e. CCBHC) or substance use facility?

The issue of medical diagnosing will be addressed in Chapter 6 in the compliance section. Specifically, there should be a clear written policy and procedure that sets forth the expectations about how medical diagnoses are to be assigned in a behavioral health setting. Keep in mind that even some psychiatrists (who are medical doctors) are not comfortable delineating the different, specific types of medical conditions such as Diabetes.

All Other Codes and Diagnoses including Neglect and Abuse, Poisoning

There are a number of other useful diagnoses and codes throughout the Tabular Index that behavioral health clinicians will need to know. A loose sampling in alphabetical order from the Tabular Index is shown in Table 3.4:

Table 3.4 Other Useful Codes for Behavioral Health Clinicians in the ICD-10-CM

Tabular Chapter	Code Blocks	Common Co-Morbid Medical Conditions or Other Conditions During a Behavioral Health Encounter
1	A00–B99	STDs, HIV, herpes, ringworm
2	C00–D49	None
3	D50–D89	None
4	E00–E89	Endocrine, nutritional and metabolic diseases
5	F01–F99	Mental, behavioral and neurodevelopmental disorders
6	G00–G99	Huntington's, Parkinson's, Alzheimer's, dementias, multiple sclerosis, seizures, migraine, sleep disorders (G-codes)
7	H00–H59	None
8	H60–H95	None
9	I00–I99	Heart disease, COPD, coronary artery disease
10	J00–J99	Asthma
11	K00–K95	None
12	L00–L99	None
13	M00–M99	None
14	N00–N99	Chronic kidney or liver failure, male/female genital disorders
15	O00–O9A	Pregnancy, pregnancy complications (alcohol, smoking), physical/sexual/psychological abuse complicating pregnancy, childbirth and the puerperium
16	P00–P96	None
17	Q00–Q99	Congenital malformations, chromosomal abnormalities (includes fetal alcohol syndrome disorder, FASD)

Tabular Chapter	Code Blocks	Common Co-Morbid Medical Conditions or Other Conditions During a Behavioral Health Encounter
18	R00–R99	Asphyxia, hypoxemia, aphagia, ataxia, R40–R46s: signs and symptoms involving cognition, perception, emotional state and behavior (suicidal and homicidal ideations), R63s: symptoms and signs concerning food and fluid intake
19	S00–T88	Poisoning, over/under dosing, toxic effects of nonmedical substances; asphyxiations (hanging, etc); adult and child abuse, neglect and other maltreatment (confirmed and suspected)
20	V00–Y99	Accidents, intentional self-harm, assaults, specific blood-alcohol levels (Y90s)
21	Z00–Z99	There are many codes/diagnoses that are applicable in Chapter 21

You may notice that there are two options for diagnosing sleep disorders in the Tabular Index, both in Chapter 5 (F-codes) and in Chapter 6 (G-codes). When the DSM-5 was released in May 2013, the authors had originally assigned the G-codes to the sleep disorders. In subsequent revisions to the text, the most recent update as of September 2016, the G-codes for sleep disorders were replaced with F-codes.

Summary

Key considerations from this chapter include:

1. While there are numerous resources available to behavioral health clinicians for accurately diagnosing and assigning code numbers to their clients, the official CMS-, HIPAA-, NCHS-, and CDC-endorsed itemization is the Tabular Index of the ICD-10-CM.
2. The burden for verifying the diagnosis code number assigned, if obtained from a source other than the Tabular Index, remains with the clinician. Do not rely on an itemization, crosswalk, EHR, the DSM series, the Internet, or other sources.
3. While there are close to 68,000 diagnoses in the Tabular Index, behavioral health clinicians will only likely utilize a small subset in their day-to-day work. This also applies to codes found in the other chapters of the Tabular Index.
4. Client safety and comprehensive healthcare service delivery will hinge on an accurate, complete, and thorough diagnostic assessment, updates,

and discharge summary. Not assigning an X-code for suicide attempts may result in an unfortunate incident, a missed opportunity, or legal ramifications.

5. It is critical that clinical decisions are made consistently with regard to some of the other diagnoses, including but not limited to the physical health codes.

Bibliography

Agency for Healthcare Research and Quality. (n.d.). *The Definition of Integrated Behavioral Health Care.* Retrieved April 1, 2016 from https://integrationacademy.ahrq.gov/atlas/What%20Is%20Integrated%20Behavioral%20Health%20Care.

American Psychiatric Association. (2015, August). *Supplement to Diagnostic and Statistical Manual of Mental Disorders*, 5th edn. Retrieved April 4, 2016 from http://dsm.psychiatryonline.org/pb-assets/dsm/update/DSM5Update2015.pdf.

Centers for Medicare & Medicaid Services. (n.d.). *FAQ 1817.* Retrieved April 3, 2016 from https://questions.cms.gov/faq.php?id=5005&faqId=1817.

Centers for Medicare & Medicaid Services. (n.d.). *FAQ 3403.* Retrieved April 3, 2016 from https://questions.cms.gov/faq.php?id=5005&faqId=3403.

Congress.gov. (2014, April 1). *PUBLIC LAW 113–93—APR. 1, 2014: Protecting Access to Medicare Act of 2014.* Retrieved April 28, 2016 from www.congress.gov/113/plaws/publ93/PLAW-113publ93.pdf.

Substance Abuse and Mental Health Services Administration. (2015). Criteria for the demonstration program to improve community mental health centers and to establish certified community behavioral health clinics, Appendix A: Quality measures and other reporting requirements. Retrieved April 4, 2016 from www.samhsa.gov/sites/default/files/programs_campaigns/ccbhc-criteria.pdf.

World Health Organization. (2016). *International Classification of Diseases, Tenth Edition, Clinical Modification (ICD-10-CM).* Retrieved April 1, 2016 from www.cdc.gov/nchs/icd/icd10cm.htm#icd2016.

Zeisset, A. (2009). ICD-10-CM enhancements: A look at the features that will improve coding accuracy. *Journal of AHIMA, 80*(2), 55–8.

Assigning Diagnoses in Behavioral Health Settings 4

In this chapter, we will look at how mental health diagnoses are typically assigned in the behavioral health industry. Specifically, we will focus on some of underpinnings of the ICD-10's CDDG and how the ICD-10 CDDG system differs from other systems in use. To briefly review: the ICD-10 CDDGs were written and published in 1992; the DSM-5 was published in 2013; and the new ICD-11 CDDGs are currently being developed to coincide with the release of ICD-11 by the WHO in 2018. When that happens, the ICD-11 CDDGs will then be the most up-to-date diagnostic manual in the world that aligns with ICD code diagnoses. For an in-depth discussion about the development of the ICD-11 CDDG, see Michael B. First et al.'s February 2015 article in *World Psychiatry*: "The development of the ICD-11 clinical descriptions and diagnostic guidelines for mental and behavioral disorders." Also, it is imperative to distinguish between the display of coded numbers and their itemized diagnoses in the ICD-10 CDDG system. To review, the ICD-10 CDDG was developed in 1992 and the ICD-10-CM (used in the USA) has been updated annually. *When you visually see code numbers in the 1992 ICD-10 CDDG, keep in mind these are not current to the US ICD-10-CM system.* Rather, we will be using the ICD-10 CDDG strictly for its utilization of arriving at diagnoses, clinical descriptions, and diagnostic criteria; therefore, the "code numbers" in the ICD-10 CDDG are outdated and clinicians are best advised to use the current year's Tabular Index.

Numerous guidelines on how to assign a diagnosis exist in the industry. Unlike those guides, this chapter will focus specifically on diagnosing with the ICD classification system, including diagnostic approach. It is acknowledged that many clinicians do use the DSM series for diagnosing behavioral health conditions. Many clinicians outside the USA also use the ICD-10 CDDG, or Blue Book, for their diagnostic criteria. This dual utilization, especially when the systems do not align, is confounding and challenging for all stakeholders, including regulatory and administrative bodies. With the publication of ICD-11, ICD-11-CM, and ICD-11 CDDG we will finally have one unified system that ends the challenges in the industry.

In the introduction to the book *A Companion to The Classification of Mental Disorders,* the authors (Cooper and Sartorius) address the fact that there are two classification systems in the world for mental and behavioral health disorders: the ICD and the DSM; they further argue that the differences historically between the ICD and DSM-IV have never been great. However, the discrepancies between the two systems became apparent when the DSM-5 was published in 2013.

The authors—originating from the UK and Switzerland respectively—distinguish between a government's position on utilization of a classification system (the ICD for example) versus a professional organization's endorsement of a classification system (the APA's DSM-5 for example). They state:

> The ICD published by the WHO must be acceptable to the governments of all the member nations and it is only published after widespread international consultations. The governments of almost all member states (including the USA) have agreed to use it. Nevertheless, whatever national governments agreed to do, professional organizations within any country are free to develop and use their own systems if they prefer and this has happened in the USA. The government of the USA uses the ICD including Chapter V, for the publication of its official health statistics, but the American Psychiatric Association has always preferred to produce—for the use of its members—its own DSM. It is quite appropriate for national classifications to exist alongside the ICD, but it is helpful to all if the reasons for this are explained and the differences between any national classifications and the ICD are listed.
>
> (Cooper & Sartorius, 2013, xvii–xviii)

Researching and studying the differences took the authors over a year to assemble and changes are ongoing as updates are made. This textbook attempts to "explain the differences" in a concise way. It is very important to consider these manuals in both a global context as well as the specific country of origin in which they are utilized. The reason the Cooper and Sartorius book is discussed here is to point out that clinicians may have two classification systems to navigate concurrently, depending on any number of variables including country of practice, philosophy, and other items.

What is important is that the clinician, provider organization, or others who are in the position of assigning clinical behavioral health diagnoses are clear and consistent in their approach to making these types of healthcare diagnoses. It would be considered best practice to have a policy and procedure that indicates which system the clinician will use to arrive at the diagnostic label that they are assigning to the case.

This chapter will also address the differences between the classification systems, with particular attention to specific diagnostic groups and diagnoses for the practicing clinician who must deal with both classification systems. Clinicians will likely be using two manuals concurrently to assign diagnoses (ICD's CDDG and DSM), until the new ICD-11 and its companion ICD-11 CDDG are published. Once the new ICD-11 and ICD-11 CDDG are published, then clinicians can exclusively use this uniform text and system, as it will provide a standardized and integrated manual created by clinicians, worldwide.

While there are differences in the two texts, they are also very much aligned. However, it is critical that behavioral health clinicians understand that the manuals do differ. Which manual or hybrid of manuals a clinician utilizes to diagnose needs to be easily articulated to justify and substantiate the diagnoses assigned. Ideally, each clinician will have a methodology for diagnosing consumers, consistent over time with reference to, and in alignment with, the already-published diagnostic classification system(s).

Behavioral Health Diagnosis: The Foundation of Treatment

Mental health diagnoses are important for a variety of reasons. They help us conceptualize the challenges a client is experiencing and they help drive the treatment planning process. Just like a physical health diagnosis, we must comprehend a person's underlying issue before we can effectively treat them. However, unlike in the medical industry, determining an exact mental health or substance use diagnosis can be more challenging, as the conditions are often not as scientifically concrete, such as blood counts or presence of infections. Arriving at a definitive mental health or substance use diagnosis can often be more of an art than a science. Diagnoses categorize individuals, label them, and are necessary for a variety of reasons. However, how accurate are mental health diagnoses, in reality? And, are codes really necessary or it is sufficient to simply understand and describe your client's experience and symptoms? Cooper and Sartorius aptly say:

> Logically, a case could be made for saying that both the ICD and DSM systems are not classifications of diagnoses, but should be called ways of identifying disorders by means of descriptive symptoms.
>
> (2013, xv)

In a typical healthcare encounter, the client will describe what they are experiencing (unless they are unconscious, impaired, or comatose); it is the behavioral health clinician's job to assimilate their own observations and data, apply any adjunct collective information, and eventually establish a diagnosis. This process is considered the first step in effective mental health treatment. In this phase of diagnosing, it is also expected that the clinician will help the client cope with, resolve, or abate the level of dysfunction or distress they are experiencing, a process that has been referred to as "The Golden Thread."

The Golden Thread is a series of related, progressive steps in the treatment of an individual that starts with the diagnostic assessment of the situation and runs through to treatment discharge. The clinical theme initially established at the assessment phase is carried through and connected to the other elements of treatment:

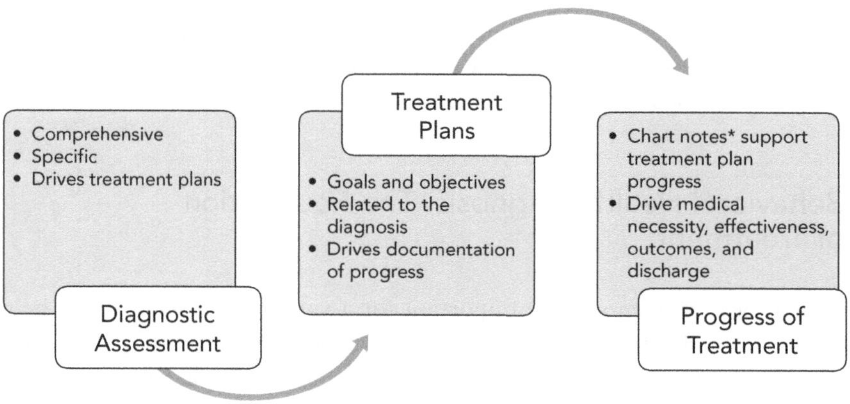

* Chart Notes, Session Notes, and Progress Notes are used interchangeably and refer to the process of documenting the problems addressed, interventions, client response to the intervention, and the plan for treatment.

The Golden Thread is the idea of taking the mental health needs and problems identified in the diagnostic assessment and then linking them to the problems to be addressed in the treatment plan. In the treatment plan, there will typically be long-term and short-term goals. The plan notes and then documents the progress of treatment for the individual, meeting and addressing the needs generated in the diagnostic assessment. In other words, the diagnosis is the "golden thread" that is driving the treatment decisions and interventions. Certainly, alleviation from, or effective management of, the distress caused by the condition/diagnosis is the ultimate goal for our work.

It has been said that the DSM manual is a good resource for early-career clinicians because the diagnostic criteria contained in the manual is highly specific. The DSM gives clear guidance as to how long and to what severity an individual must experience symptoms before the client can be diagnosed with a certain condition. The third-party payers in the USA rely on these classifications and criteria to determine if a diagnosis is reimbursable or if a diagnosis needs more specification.

It has been said that the ICD-10's CDDG manual is a good resource for more experienced clinicians who feel competent enough to "practice the art of diagnosing." As we learned in Chapter 1, the 1992 ICD-10 CDDG provides less specific, time-driven diagnostic criteria and thresholds. As a result, the diagnostic process really does come down to the clinician's judgment as to whether or not the client has crossed the clinical threshold.

The function of delineating the two diagnostic classification systems (ICD and DSM) is to help educate the clinician about their clinical diagnostic description options. Once the new ICD-11 CDDGs are published, we will then have a worldwide, standardized, single uniform classification system. Some argue that the world movement towards a uniform diagnostic system with the ICD-11 may also positively impact our practitioner's cultural competence understanding and practices.

Until the ICD-11 CDDG is published, however, it is imperative that practitioners do the following:

- Learn both systems and make an evaluation as to which one (or both) they will utilize
- Develop a standardized approach for assigning diagnoses to clients
- Explain to the client how they have arrived at the client's diagnosis, and how that diagnosis impacts them both clinically and administratively
- Compose a policy and procedure that outline how diagnoses will be assigned for compliance and audit purposes

Clinical Applications of the Systems: Notable Clinical Differences Between the DSM-5 and ICD-10 CDDG

As discussed briefly in Chapter 1, the DSM-5 is quite different from its DSM predecessors. With its publication, along with the mandated shift to use ICD-10-CM codes for diagnoses in the USA, the use of both systems has put clinicians in a difficult position:

> If we are mandated to use the ICD-10 CM codes, which diagnostic classification system do we then utilize to support and substantiate the assigned ICD-10-CM diagnosis? Moreover, what do we do if the clinical criteria thresholds to meet certain diagnoses are quite different between the two systems?
>
> (Author's own words, 2015)

There is no easy answer to this dilemma of negotiating between two manuals with the exception of the eventual publication of the ICD-11 CDDG (remember, this is not expected to happen until at least 2018 or much later), depending on when the WHO approves the new ICD-11 and the USA then adopts its own version of the ICD-11 (called the ICD-11-CM). Additionally, clinicians may find they prefer one manual over the other, depending on the diagnostic category or even access to financial resources to support the DSM.

Language Differences Between the ICD and DSM Systems

There are some critical language differences between the DSM-5 and the ICD-10 CDDG. Keep in mind the ICD-10 CDDG was published in 1992 and many terms may now be pejorative or simply obsolete. It is certainly expected that the ICD-11 CDDG will bring an updated use of language to the clinical criteria. Below are some examples of the language and diagnostic category differences:

DSM-5	ICD-10*
Substance Use Disorders	Substance Abuse, Dependence
Autism Spectrum Disorder	Asperger's
Disruptive Mood Dysregulation Disorder	No comparable diagnosis (except in USA)

DSM-5	ICD-10*
Hoarding Disorder	No comparable diagnosis (except in USA)
Binge-Eating Disorder	No comparable diagnosis (except in USA)
Intellectual/Neurocognitive Disorders	Mental retardation
No stand-alone Mania conditions	Entire diagnostic category of Mania
One Schizophrenia diagnosis	Many Schizophrenia diagnoses

*There are also some differences between the ICD-10-CM Tabular Index used in the USA and the 1992 ICD-10 CDDG. Terms displayed above are terms generally used when utilizing the entire ICD-10 system. As of this writing, some of the new DSM-5 diagnoses are being proposed for inclusion in the ICD-11 but final determination will not be made until the WHO Assembly officially approves the ICD-11.

The remainder of this chapter will focus on the clinical criteria differences between the ICD-10 CDDG and the DSM-5. It is critical that practitioners understand the diagnostic criteria referenced in order to substantiate their diagnoses in their documentation. There are some significant differences between the DSM-5, ICD-10 CDDG, and ICD-10-CM codes. The differences will be discussed according to diagnostic categories:

1. Substance Use Disorders
2. Schizophrenia and Psychotic Disorders
3. Anxiety, Trauma, and Adjustment Disorders
4. Mood Disorders
5. Childhood Disorders
6. Other Notable Disorders.

Substance Use Disorders

The DSM-5 completely reorganized the Substance Use category from its predecessors. Previous versions of the DSM listed Substance *Abuse* and Substance *Dependence* as two main categories of diagnosing the severity of a person's chemical use. However, the DSM-5 has now split the Substances into two general diagnostic categories: *Substance Use* Disorder and *Substance-Induced* Disorders. A further distinguishing factor is assigning a Mild, Moderate, or Severe-use specifier designation to the new DSM-5 diagnosis, and this is driven by the number of criteria and symptoms the client is experiencing. Taken alone, the DSM-5 protocol is straightforward and works well as it is based on the premise that substance use disorders can have a range of implications and the severity is to be assigned based on a dimensional approach, which makes sense. The disconnect between the DSM-5 and the ICD-series is the fact that the ICD series retains the categorization of Substance Abuse and Dependence. This is where the confusion, the coding numbers, and the ability to cross-reference the DSM-5 and the ICD series become untenable for the clinician.

Keep in mind that a clinician may need to use both classification systems concurrently, for the same case, for different purposes. For example, a prior authorization for services form request may ask for a DSM-5 diagnosis and corresponding diagnostic criteria where, for billing and claims, we must use the ICD-10-CM in order to be compliant for HIPAA purposes.

In the article, "Disorders related to use of psychoactive substances in DSM-5: Changes and challenges," in the *Indian Journal of Psychological Medicine*, the authors (Bhad et al.) in their commentary indicate that:

> One of the most significant changes in [the] new classification system is abolition of substance dependence and abuse as separate categories. This change has addressed the debate on whether abuse and dependence are separate disorders or are on a continuum . . . The decision to shift to a single diagnostic category of substance use disorder in lieu of separate categories for abuse and dependence is rooted in the one of basic guiding principle for DSM-5 that is to shift from stringent categorical approach to dimensional approach.
>
> (Bhad et al., 2015, 470–2)

Aside from the dimensional versus categorical conceptualization of substances and other disorders, we encounter another discrepancy with the Substance Use Disorders between classification systems: the discrepancy between the two manuals in the actual number of diagnoses available between them. We are already aware that the ICD-10-CM has greatly expanded the number of available diagnoses from approximately 14,000 to 68,000 (see Chapter 1). Table 4.1 demonstrates the differences in the substances between the ICD-10-CM and the DSM-5:

Table 4.1 DSM-IV-TR to Number of Substance Use Diagnoses in the DSM-5 versus the ICD-10-CM

DSM-IV-TR CODE Dependence/Abuse	DSM-5: Codes and # of Diagnoses	DESCRIPTION (ICD-10-CM) by Substance	ICD-10-CM OPTIONS: Codes and # of Diagnoses
303.9; 305	F10s: 8	Alcohol	F10s: 47
304; 305.5	F11s: 10	Opioids	F11s: 41
304.3; 305.2	F12s: 10	Cannabis	F12s: 34
304.1; 305.4	F13s: 8	Sedative, hypnotic, or anxiolytics	F13s: 52
304.2; 305.6	F14s: 10	Cocaine	F14s: 44
304.4; 305.7	F15s: 10	Other stimulants	F15s: 45
304.5; 305.3	F16s: 8	Hallucinogens	F16s: 38
305.1	F17s: 4	Nicotine	F17s: 20
304.6; 305.9	F18s: 6	Inhalants	F18s: 37
304.9; 305.9	F19s: 7	Other psychoactive substance related disorders	F19s: 57

The following graphic makes a similar demonstration of the differences in substance use diagnoses between the ICD-10-CM and the DSM-5:

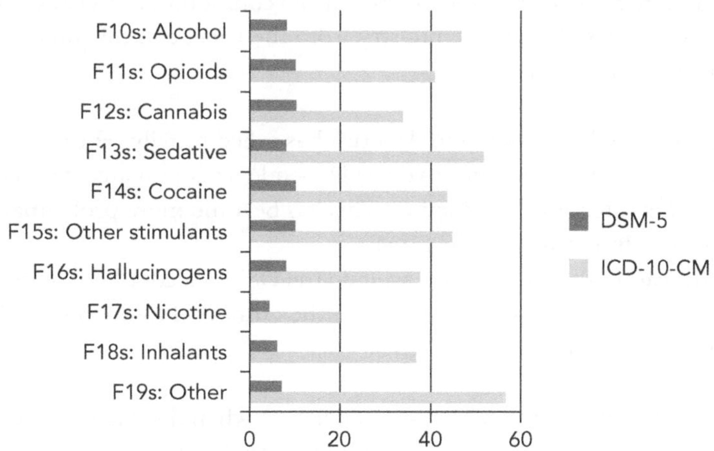

So, between the two manuals, we have differences in:

- the number of available diagnoses in each manual with the ICD-10-CM giving us many more options than the DSM-5;
- the language, or title, of the actual diagnosis name ("Abuse" or "Dependence" versus "Use" or "Induced");
- diagnostic criteria differences and thresholds between the DSM-5 and the ICD-10 CDDG.

The diagnostic criteria differences between the manuals are most notable when you visually compare the diagnostic guidelines in the ICD-10 CDDG to those in the DSM-5. For example, the ICD-10 CDDG does not differentiate between the substances (e.g. alcohol, cocaine, or cannabis). Instead, the diagnostic criteria itemize the *states* that the client struggles with, such as: Acute Intoxication, Harmful Use (aka Abuse), Dependence Syndrome, Withdrawal State, Withdrawal State with Delirium, Psychotic Disorder, Amnesic Syndrome, and Residual and Late-Onset Psychotic Disorder.

In contrast, the DSM-5 itemizes the diagnostic criteria by the *substance*: Alcohol-Related Disorders or Opioid-Related Disorders, for example. The most effective way to understand the clinical criteria differences is to visually compare the Substance-Related and Addictive Disorders in the DSM-5 versus the diagnostic categories and criteria for psychoactive substances in the ICD-10 CDDG (pages 70–83). It is recommended that clinicians have a standardized, consistent approach to diagnosing and coding these disorders.

Finally, there are other differences that can confound a clinician working in the Substance Use Disorders industry from the legal, clinical and prevalence perspective. For example:

- **Legal:** The legal system in America has relied heavily on the distinction between Substance Abuse versus Dependence and many state laws still use this categorical distinction. This has become more problematic with the new framework in the DSM-5
- **Clinical:** In the study "How well do the DSM-5 alcohol use designations map to the ICD-10-CM disorders?" the authors (Hoffmann and Kopak, 2015) noted the following items:

    - The DSM-5 and ICD-10-CM align best when the diagnoses are either "no diagnosis" or a *severe* substance use diagnosis is given.
    - However, slightly more than one-third (35.9%) of patients given a *mild* substance use designation under the DSM-5 would not receive

a diagnosis under the ICD-10-CM, and 1.5% of DSM-5 *moderate* patients would not receive a diagnosis based on the ICD-10-CM.

- **Prevalence of Substance Use Disorders using DSM-5 only:** There is an increased possibility of over-diagnosing substance use disorders in the younger individuals who have "occasional harmful substance use."

Class Discussion

What are some of the challenges you can anticipate regarding the differences between the ICD series and DSM series in the Substance Use Disorder section?

Which area (legal, clinical, or prevalence) might be most impacted by the differences in the manuals and what are the implications for this?

What are the advantages/disadvantages to having more diagnoses available in ICD-10-CM versus fewer in DSM-5?

What other concerns as a practicing clinician might you have regarding the manual differences in the Substance Use categories?

Schizophrenia and Psychotic Disorders

This diagnostic category presents a number of dilemmas for the clinician. As you read in Chapter 1, there is one code number for Schizophrenia listed in the DSM-5 and there are several available codes for differing types of Schizophrenia in the ICD-10-CM. For those using an EHR, it is very important to ensure that all the Schizophrenia types in the ICD-10-CM codes are available for use. In fact, simply using the DSM-5 code (F20.9 Schizophrenia, Unspecified) has been met with rejections by some payers such as CMS until very recently, creating undue financial hardship for providers. Provider organizations, not understanding the differences between the DSM-5 and the ICD-10-CM had been caught off guard by this CMS action. CMS follows the ICD-10-CM rules and guidelines and expects their provider organizations (and clinicians) to do the same. This is a legitimate position especially in light of the fact that the ICD-10-CM lists all the varieties of Schizophrenia.

With regard to the actual diagnosis of schizophrenia, the rationale given for the elimination of the schizophrenia subtypes in the DSM-5 is best explained by a very thorough paper titled, "Definition and description of schizophrenia in the DSM-5" by Tandon et al. (2013) in *Schizophrenia Research*:

> The classic DSM-IV subtypes of schizophrenia provide a poor description of the heterogeneity of schizophrenia, have low diagnostic stability, do not exhibit distinctive patterns of treatment response or longitudinal course, and are not heritable. Except for the paranoid and undifferentiated subtypes, other subtypes are rarely diagnosed. As a result, these subtypes of schizophrenia were eliminated from DSM-5.

Carefully review the illustration below:

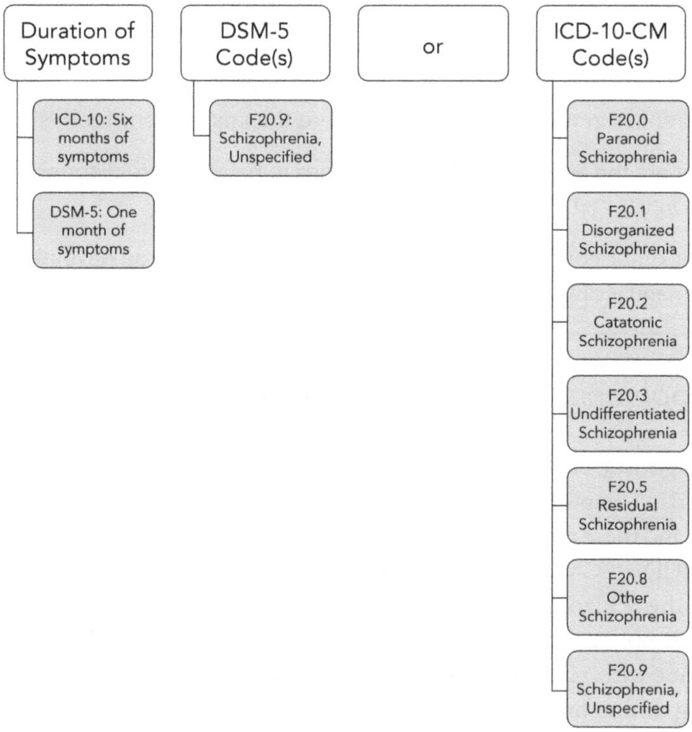

One of the biggest differences between the ICD and the DSM comes from the length of time, or duration, that a client must exhibit symptoms before the diagnosis can be given. In the DSM-5, the duration is a period of *one* month whereas the duration in the ICD-10 CDDG states *six* months. This difference between the manuals is significant; and it is therefore hoped by many in the behavioral health field that the new ICD-11 CDDG will bring these discrepancies into alignment, or at least provide one consistent, standardized approach to diagnosing Schizophrenia (i.e. by exclusively using the ICD series).

> **Class Discussion**
>
> Which system, the DSM or the ICD, has a better understanding of the Schizophrenic condition? What are the pros and cons of each?

From an EHR point of view, any narrative notation of a schizophrenic subtype will be missed when using the DSM-5 code for Schizophrenia, F20.9. This absence of specificity could affect Clinical Decision Support (CDS) rules, automatically-linked patient education materials, or have other implications. Decision support rules are computer code written into your EHR system that gives you an alert when there is something to be concerned about. For example, you could set up the EHR to fire a CDS rule that reminds you to check lithium levels every six months based on a person's diagnosis and last set of lab results in the EHR. Keep in mind that some EHR vendors have obtained their ICD-10-CM codes directly from the APA. Because of the revisions to this category, only one code will populate in the drop downs in those EHRs: F20.9 Schizophrenia, Unspecified. As we saw from Chapter 2, the utilization of Unspecified can be potentially problematic. Additionally, the ICD-10-CM Tabular Index gives us many choices for this condition, and it would be appropriate to diagnose the most specific form of Schizophrenia if the client meets the criteria in the ICD-10 CDDG.

In terms of other Psychotic Disorders, the subtle differences are difficult to see except when they are placed in a side-by-side comparison:

Psychotic Disorder in the ICD-10-CM Tabular Index	Psychotic Disorder in the DSM-5
F21: Schizotypal Disorder	F21: Schizotypal **Personality** Disorder
F22: Delusional Disorders	F22: Delusional Disorder
F24: Shared Psychotic Disorder	
F28: Other psychotic disorder not due to a substance or known physiological condition	F28: Other specified schizophrenia spectrum and other psychotic disorder
F29: Unspecified psychosis not due to a substance or known physiological condition	F29: Unspecified schizophrenia spectrum and other psychotic disorder

It behooves the clinician to know what the differences are between the systems and to develop a standardized, consistent approach to assessing and diagnosing schizophrenia and psychotic disorders.

Anxiety, Trauma, and Adjustment Disorders

In the Anxiety Disorder category, one of the most distinctive differences between the DSM and the ICD involves the duration of symptoms. In order to diagnose a consumer with a certain condition, they must have "x (number of) symptoms" for a certain duration or period of time in order to meet the threshold and diagnostic criteria for that diagnosis. Much as we saw with regard to schizophrenia, some of the time differences between the classification systems are notable. To best illustrate this, Table 4.2 outlines the duration of symptom differences between the DSM-5 and the ICD-10 CDDG:

Table 4.2 Duration of Anxiety Symptoms Needed for Diagnosis

Common Diagnosis Name	ICD-10's CDDG (Blue Book)	DSM-6
Agoraphobia	No timeframe, clinical judgment	Symptoms for 6 months
Social Phobia	No timeframe, clinical judgment	Symptoms for 6 months
Generalized Anxiety Disorder	Symptoms for "several months"	Symptoms for 6 months
OCD	Symptoms for "at least 2 weeks"	No timeframe given
Post-Traumatic Stress Disorder	"Evidence PTSD arose within 6 months of a traumatic event"	No timeframe given

In addition to the timeframe differences, a few other noteworthy contrasts exist, including:

- Hoarding Disorder is only present in the DSM-5 and in the US version of the ICD-10-CM. It may / may not be included in the upcoming ICD-11 that is used internationally.
- Obsessive Compulsive Disorder (OCD) has its own chapter in the DSM-5 whereas OCD is contained in the Anxiety section of the Tabular Index.
- The ICD-10-CM Tabular Index itemizes more specific phobias than the DSM-5; in other words, with the ICD-10-CM you have more specific choices that accurately represent the phobias.

The diagnosis of Post-Traumatic Stress Disorder (PTSD) deserves special attention due to its clinical prevalence across the globe. The DSM-5 separated out the Trauma and Stressor-Related Disorders by giving them their own chapter. But there are some challenges with this approach, especially as it relates to PTSD, as Table 4.3 illustrates. The DSM-5 gives us one possible code number for PTSD, and it does not differentiate between the three types of PTSD listed in the ICD-10-CM, in terms of coding numbers. In fact, F43.10 is linked to an "unspecified" diagnosis and we know that over-utilization of unspecified diagnoses can cause complications. The ICD-10 CDDGs do not specify, define, or delineate between the conditions of "acute" or "chronic" and clinicians will therefore have to develop a standard protocol and definition for these specifiers. As of July 2016, the DSM-5 still lists only one diagnosis for PTSD, F43.10.

Table 4.3 Availability of PTSD Codes in the ICD-10-CM versus the DSM-5

PTSD in the ICD-10 CM	PTSD in the DSM-5
F43.10 Post-Traumatic Stress Disorder, Unspecified	F43.10 Post-Traumatic Stress Disorder
F43.11 Post-Traumatic Stress Disorder, Acute	(Subtypes and specifiers apply, but do not have an associated coding number. You would notate this in the narrative portion of the medical record, which can be missed by not reading the text portion of the record.)
F43.12 Post-Traumatic Stress Disorder, Chronic	

Shortly after go-live of the ICD-10-CM in the USA in October 2015, many third-party payers were requiring that any diagnosis of F43.10 PTSD, Unspecified be defined as either acute or chronic, and the unspecified code was getting rejected for its lack of specificity. As a result, it is important to establish a strong clinical policy to enable clinicians to differentiate between acute or chronic conditions, and to provide agency-wide consistency.

The DSM-5 specifier for PTSD (acute versus chronic) is captured in the text narrative portion of the medical record, not as a discrete data element that can be easily extracted or shared with others through health information technology (i.e. a code number such as F43.11 or F43.12). Chapter 1 addressed this situation that affects certain disorders, including PTSD, as being potentially problematic to standardized and effective use of EHRs.

Adjustment Disorders were placed in the Trauma and Stressor-Related Disorders section of the DSM-5 because one of the hallmark criteria is "*symptoms in response to an identifiable stressor.*" The ICD-10-CM Tabular Index itemizes the different Adjustment Disorders right after the PTSD category, in the Anxiety section. Of particular note is the duration of symptom differences between the DSM-5 and the ICD-10 CDDG. The ICD-10 CDDG states a person must exhibit symptoms for a period of *"3 months or longer"* before they can be diagnosed with one of the Adjustment Disorders. The DSM-5, on the other hand, indicates a very strict timeframe for Adjustment Disorders: *occurring within 3 months and lasting no longer than 6 months.* This is one of the best examples of an exact timeframe in the DSM-5 in comparison to the ICD-10's CDDG which exhibits more flexibility.

Acute Stress Disorder (DSM-5) and Acute Stress Reaction (ICD-10 CDDG) are assigned the same diagnostic code (F43.0) in the ICD-10-CM Tabular Index. However, significant differences exist between the diagnostic clinical criteria for this disorder across the two manuals. The illustration below highlights the timeframe differences between the two:

DSM-5 Acute Stress Disorder

- Symptoms: "typically begin immediately after the trauma, but persistence for at least 3 days and up to a month"
- Duration: 3 days to 1 month

ICD-10 CDDG Acute Stress Reaction

- Symptoms: "usually appear within a few minutes . . . and disappear within 2–3 days"
- Duration: immediate to 3 days

As always with documentation, it is imperative to notate the *duration* as well as the *number* and *severity* of symptoms the client is reporting to substantiate the diagnosis. If your protocol is to use one manual over the other, then it is important to know the differences.

We have seen that using the diagnosis category "unspecified" can cause challenges for a variety of reasons. There are a few diagnoses in the Anxiety category that have a general code number assigned to them in the DSM-5 that actually map to an equivalent diagnosis, but remain at the "unspecified" level in the ICD-10-CM. It is an important reminder of the importance of assigning the "most specific code available" (delineated in Chapter 2 on the coding and documentation rules and guidelines). For example, the diagnosis of Agoraphobia has subtle, but critical, differences between the manuals in terms of code numbers and conditions. Table 4.4 outlines these differences:

Table 4.4 Difference Between DSM-5 and ICD-10-CM, Agoraphobia

Code Number	DSM-5 Diagnosis Name	ICD-10-CM Diagnosis Name
F40.00	Agoraphobia	Agoraphobia, Unspecified
F40.01		Agoraphobia, with Panic Disorder
F40.02		Agoraphobia, without Panic Disorder

Class Discussion

What is the difference between the three ICD-10-CM diagnoses of Agoraphobia and how do you make that distinction? Would there ever be a situation that you would use "Unspecified?" If yes, when?

Tables 4.5 and 4.6 depict additional Anxiety diagnoses that differ across the classification systems:

Table 4.5 Difference Between DSM-5 and ICD-10-CM, Social Phobia

Code Number	DSM-5 Diagnosis Name	ICD-10-CM Diagnosis Name
F40.10	Social Anxiety Disorder (Social Phobia)	Social Phobia, Unspecified
F40.11		Social Phobia, Generalized

Table 4.6 Difference Between DSM-5 and ICD-10-CM, Panic Disorder

Code Number	DSM-5 Diagnosis Name	ICD-10-CM Diagnosis Name
F41.0	Panic Disorder	Panic Disorder (episodic paroxysmal anxiety) without agoraphobia

Mood Disorders

There are a number of differences between the ICD-10-CM, ICD-10 CDDG and DSM-5 that will be discussed in this section. A major difference occurs in the Bipolar category. In addition, the other major mood disorder diagnoses will be outlined as well as the time frame differences in the two manuals.

The Bipolar sections in both the ICD-10-CM and the DSM-5 are quite thorough. At a high level, the major differences are:

1. The DSM-5 uses the terms: "Bipolar I" and "Bipolar II."
2. The ICD-10-CM utilizes the categories of: Manic Episodes, Bipolar Disorder, and Bipolar Disorder II. The term "Bipolar I" is not used in the ICD-10-CM and some may find this confounding.

Across the manuals and classification systems, the three defining mood states have common ground: Mania, Hypomania, and Major Depression. However, it is only in the ICD-10-CM system that the clinician will find the entire block of F30 codes, which are Manic Episodes. For example, if an individual has a manic episode only, without the depressive cycle, it seems that using the F30 code might be the most appropriate diagnosis to assign. While this seems relatively straightforward, it creates a dilemma for clinicians in that the DSM-5 does not contain any F30-block diagnoses. In fact, the DSM-5 suggests that if a client has presented with only a manic episode, it is most likely that the individual will *"experience major depressive episodes during the course of their lives."* The diagnostic criteria to meet the F30 diagnoses in the ICD-10-CM can be found in the ICD-10 CDDG, and this diagnosis can certainly be applied to certain cases.

This variation has the potential to be confusing to clinicians, especially when they see a client who has only experienced a manic episode to date. Understanding when to diagnose what disorder, especially when it comes to the differences between the manuals, will be an area for further explication and training.

Two other differences need to be pointed out. Table 4.7 shows the differences in the naming conventions across the systems. Another potential point of confusion is the fact that the DSM-5 does not contain any diagnoses in the F30 category (Manic Episodes) but they are available and legitimate diagnoses in the ICD-10-CM. Clinical guidance and policies need to be developed to help clinicians understand what is expected of them.

Table 4.7 Naming Differences in Bipolar Between the DSM-5 and ICD-10-CM

Code Block	DSM-5 Naming Convention	ICD-10-CM Naming Convention
F30s		Manic Episodes
F31s	Bipolar I Disorder	Bipolar Disorder
F31.81	Bipolar II Disorder	Bipolar II Disorder

Major Depressive Disorder, either Single Episode or Recurrent Episodes, are addressed in both the ICD-10 CDDG and the DSM-5 and, for the most part, are aligned in terms of the diagnoses and code numbers. The diagnostic criteria are very similar to each other in each classification system, with one major exception: the actual hallmark criteria of a major depressive episode.

For example, in the DSM-5, the two hallmark criteria cited are: 1. Depressed mood most of the day, or 2. Loss of interest and pleasure. In order to give a Major Depression diagnosis per the DSM-5, one or both of these hallmark criteria are required. However, in the ICD-10 CDDG, there are three hallmark criteria: 1. Depressed mood most of the day, or 2. Loss of interest and pleasure, or 3. Reduced energy leading to increased fatigability and diminished activity.

Class Discussion

What hallmark criteria for Major Depression are most important? How would you manage the diagnosing of an individual with Major Depression if the criteria were not met per the DSM-5, but the individual did meet the criteria per the ICD-10 CDDG? What would you do?

Many clients with major depressions engage in self-harm behaviors, up to and including suicide attempts. It is therefore incumbent upon behavioral health clinicians to code for, document, and notate these acts of self-harm. In addition, the ICD-10 CDDG clearly endorses this practice standard:

> Acts of self-harm associated with mood disorders . . . should be recorded by means of an additional code from Chapter XX of ICD-10.

One significant benefit of having the entire Tabular Index of diagnoses, conditions, and syndromes from which to choose can be seen when we examine the inclusion of self-harm codes, ranging from X71-X83, in the ICD-10-CM Tabular Index. In our current approach to mental health, where the use of technology (EHRs) to track our clients' diagnoses and treatment for collaboration of care is the norm, it is imperative for clinicians to code for the intentional self-harm in the EHR. More specifically, if a client is demonstrating self-harm tendencies or behaviors and it is not coded, then other providers may miss this crucial detail. Furthermore, this assignment of specific X71–X83 self-harm codes is essential because it enables the providers to identify and treat a pattern of increasing severity in self-harm methods. Without this specificity, crucial aspects of the case could be missed, which could potentially have devastating effects on the client's treatment and mental health. Finally, securing clinical charting documentation that is highly descriptive in nature can also yield more comprehensive results in the areas of research on population health statistics and suicide prevention efforts. The importance of coding and documentation of the X-codes in our industry cannot be overemphasized.

Disruptive Mood Dysregulation Disorder (DMDD) is a new DSM-5 diagnosis that is currently not included in the ICD-10 CDDG or in the WHO's ICD-10. Clinical criteria can only be obtained via the DSM-5 at this point in time. That may eventually change with the updated ICD CDDGs.

Generally speaking, the ICD-10 CDDG gives some lenience and room for the clinician to decide *when* to assign a Major Depressive diagnosis. For example, while the criteria indicate that most symptom durations will be *"of at least 2 weeks,"* the CDDG adds that *"shorter periods may be reasonable if symptoms are unusually severe and of rapid onset,"* leaving room for clinical judgment. This is another example of how the ICD-10 CDDG gives the clinician room to "practice the art of diagnosing."

The severity levels for a diagnosis of a Major Depression between the two classification systems is also important to note. The ICD-10 CDDG is actually a bit more specific in the number of required symptoms and durations than the DSM-5. Specifically, the differences are shown in Table 4.8:

Table 4.8 Severity Levels of Major Depression Between the DSM-5 and ICD-10 CDDG

ICD-10	**DSM-5 (page 188)**
Mild: At least 2 typical symptoms + 2 others*	Mild: Few, if any symptoms
Moderate: 2 or 3 symptoms + 3 preferably 4 others	Moderate: Number of symptoms are between mild and severe
Severe: All 3 typical symptoms + at least 4 others	Severe: In excess of that which is required to make the diagnosis

*Symptoms are listed on page 119 of the ICD-10 CDDG.

Finally, there is a notable timeframe difference between the two systems pertaining to the diagnosis of Cyclothymia. In the DSM-5, the duration of symptoms for adults is *"for at least two years"* whereas the ICD-10 CDDG does not issue a time frame for meeting the diagnostic threshold.

Other Notable Differences

This section will discuss the other behavioral health diagnoses that have notable clinical differences between the two classification systems or code number inconsistencies that impact both clinicians and revenue cycles.

Eating Disorders

Eating Disorders is a complex clinical landscape that is confusing across the manuals. First, Binge-Eating Disorder was in the DSM-5 but not present in the ICD-10-CM for a period of two years. Despite regulatory updates, this diagnostic category remains confusing between the DSM and ICD-series. Let us look at Table 4.9 to see the differences visually between the manuals:

DSM-5 Name	DSM-5 Code(s)	ICD-10-CM Name	ICD-10-CM Code(s)
		Anorexia Nervosa, Unspecified	F50.00
Anorexia Nervosa, Restricting Type	F50.01	Anorexia Nervosa, Restricting Type	F50.01
Anorexia Nervosa, Binge-Eating/Purging Type	F50.02	Anorexia Nervosa, Binge-Eating/Purging Type	F50.02
Bulimia Nervosa	F50.2	Bulimia Nervosa	F50.2
Binge-Eating Disorder	F50.81	Binge-Eating Disorder	F50.81
Other Specified Feeding or Eating Disorder	F50.89	Other Eating Disorders	F50.89
Pica, in Adults	F50.89		
Avoidant/Restrictive Food Intake Disorder	F50.89		
Unspecified Feeding or Eating Disorder	F50.9	Eating Disorder, Unspecified	F50.9

Note that the DSM-5 diagnosis Rumination Disorder is purposely not included in the above table.

F50.89 in the DSM-5 represents three different diagnoses, which can lead to confusion when looking at claims data and provider profiling. Let us consider the implications and possible challenges to these scenarios:

- The code on the claim form for purposes of payment reimbursement is an "other" code that may cause a delayed claim, denial, or question about "why isn't a more specific diagnosis assigned?"
- In the DSM-5, F50.89 has been assigned to three different diagnoses: Avoidant/restrictive food intake disorder, Other specified feeding or eating disorder, and Pica, in adults. Looking at the code number alone, it will be uncertain which diagnosis was actually intended unless the narrative portion of the medical record is reviewed.
- Finally, Anorexia Nervosa must be typed in the DSM-5 into *either* restricting *or* binge-eating/purging type. There is no option for Anorexia, Unspecified in the DSM-5 but there is in the ICD-10-CM (F50.00).

Childhood Disorders

The new DSM-5 has removed the section "Disorders Usually First Diagnosed in Infancy, Childhood, or Adolescence." Instead of isolating these diagnoses into one section in the book, the DSM-5 authors incorporate them into the corresponding diagnostic category and typically list them first. From a clinical perspective, not grouping the Childhood Disorders in one place enables the clinician to isolate a diagnosis category first. In comparison, the ICD-10-CM retains the childhood and adolescent category in the F90–F98 block of the Tabular Index.

There are some notable differences between the classification systems that child and adolescent clinicians will need to keep in mind. The first is that the ICD-10 CDDG as well as the WHO's ICD-10 use the term "Hyperkinetic" to describe Attention-Deficit Hyperactivity. Clinicians in the USA may not be used to seeing this word, and yet it does represent Attention-Deficit Hyperactivity. The F90.X codes in the WHO's ICD-10 version and the ICD-10 CDDG are labeled as "Hyperkinetic Disorders" but in the ICD-10-CM used in the USA they are called "Attention-Deficit Hyperactivity Disorders."

The second difference is in the conduct-disorder category, i.e. the F91.X section, "Conduct Disorders." Most of the Conduct Disorders are aligned between the DSM-5. The ICD-10-CM F91.0, "Conduct Disorder confined to family context" is exclusive to the ICD series, which can be quite helpful to clinicians.

Table 4.10 shows some subtle differences between the DSM-5 and ICD-10-CM in the following diagnosis categories: Disinhibited Social Engagement Disorder and Provisional Tic Disorder. The rationale for pointing these out is twofold: first, the subtle differences may impact the case formulation of a client; second, clinical documentation will also be impacted as supporting the submitted ICD-10-CM diagnoses for HIPAA purposes will need to be present. Note the difference in the names of the diagnoses, per category:

Table 4.10 Social Engagement and Provisional Tics Disorders Differences

Code Number	DSM-5	ICD-10-CM
F94.2	Disinhibited social engagement disorder	Disinhibited attachment disorder of childhood
F95.0	Provisional tic disorder	Transient tic disorder

Pervasive Developmental Disorders, F80–F89

The DSM-5 now has a diagnosis called Autism Spectrum Disorder (ASD) that has been seen by some to be "a new, more accurate, and medically and scientifically useful way of diagnosing individuals with autism-related disorders."

In contrast, the ICD-10-CM contains the varied autism-related disorders that many clinicians are accustomed to: autistic disorder, Retts syndrome, other childhood disintegrative disorders, Asperger's syndrome, and other pervasive developmental disorders. Asperger's is no longer a separate, coded diagnosis in the new DSM-5; instead, a clinician would have to utilize the ASD diagnosis as recommended by the DSM-5 and APA. From a coding and documentation standpoint, this brings up several potential complications:

- The code number F84.0 represents "Autism Spectrum Disorder" in the DSM-5 and concurrently "Autistic Disorder" in the ICD-10-CM. Is there a difference between Autism Spectrum Disorder and Autistic Disorder? Asperger's retains its individual code (F84.5) in the ICD-10-CM. What if you determined that Asperger's was the most appropriate diagnosis for your client, but you are being asked to submit a diagnosis and code *only from* the DSM-5 (i.e. prior authorization)? Unless there is a written text narrative or accompaniment to your submission, the receiver of this information would only see the DSM-5 coded numerical value of F84.0, Autism Spectrum Disorder.
- The discrepancy between DSM's ASD and the ICD's Autism (both coded as F84.0) is a challenge and confusing for providers and clients. Some third parties initially denied coverage for F84.0, Autistic Disorder showing on claims, and yet the clinician really was coding for ASD, per the DSM-5.
- Some payer entities in the USA have indicated that they will only reimburse certain diagnoses IF they are contained in the DSM-5 manual. The

DSM-5 clearly states that those individuals previously diagnosed in the DSM-IV as having Asperger's "should (now) be given the diagnosis of ASD." Some of the complications for this dilemma are:

- Time and staff resources are needed both for understanding the discrepancy and for explaining the discrepancy to the claims reviewer, utilization management department, or on the prior authorization form.
- The client with Asperger's would like to know why they were given a DSM-5 diagnosis of Autism Spectrum Disorder but the medical record and claims data in the third-party repository reflects a diagnosis of Autistic Disorder.
- The DSM-5 assigns three specifiers to ASD based on a number of dimensional factors. There is one code number, F84.0. If you are reviewing the Diagnostic history tab in an EHR, would you be able to see how severe this client's diagnosis is by looking at the code number only? What would you have to do to understand what level of severity the client has with DSM-5's Autism Spectrum Disorder?

Assigning Diagnoses in ICD-10-CM Outside of Chapter 5's F-Codes

The ICD-10-CM has a plethora of diagnoses to choose from in addition to the codes from Chapter 5, the Mental and Behavioral Disorders section. Largely due to healthcare reform, behavioral health clinicians are now faced with the numerous concerns our consumers bring into the office. Contributing factors to a person's behavioral health condition can include:

- physical health issues: genetic, metabolic, acute and chronic conditions;
- other conditions that affect behavioral health of consumers:
    - stressors or other contributing factors that influence behavioral health;
    - toxic effects and blood levels;
    - external causes contributing to the clinical picture and diagnostic assessment.

A section titled the "Annex" exists near the end of the ICD-10 CDDG; here, the WHO outlines any number of contributory factors that are "often associated with mental and behavioral disorders." What the ICD-10 CDDG does not provide is the clinical criteria or diagnostic guidelines to actually assign some of these codes. Keep in mind, as discussed in Chapter 2, that there are certain instances where the clinician must "Code First" the underlying etiology of a presenting problem or diagnosis. Both the DSM-5 and the ICD-10-CM endorse this practice so it may be confusing to clinicians about how and when to apply these additional codes.

The best answer to this challenge is for the clinician to have a standardized approach to assigning diagnoses, encapsulated in a written clinical guideline, policy, or procedure. For example, some agencies may recommend X while others may prefer Y. It is also important for the clinician to diagnose all known, contributory factors to the presenting problem in their initial intake session. To do this properly, the clinician must know and understand all available codes contained in the ICD-10-CM.

Physical Health Codes

Ensuring accurate coding and documentation for co-morbid health conditions is critical to any effective healthcare delivery system. From a Health Information Technology (HIT) perspective, it is not sufficient to simply write down a contributory medical condition in the text narrative portion of the record. For research, epidemiology, data collection, integrated care, population health, and statistical purposes, we must code *all applicable* conditions that affect the client and their current health status.

With the removal of the multi-axial system in the DSM-5, clinicians are instructed to combine the old Axis III (medical conditions) with Axes I and II:

> Clinicians should continue to list medical conditions that are important to the understanding or management of an individual's mental disorder(s).
> (American Psychiatric Association, 2013, 16)

We will look at the most common physical health diseases linked to serious mental illness and/or psychotropic medication treatments as identified in the article "Physical illness in patients with severe mental disorders. I. Prevalence, impact of medications and disparities in health care," by De Hert et al. in *World Psychiatry*.

In addition, we will look at certain metabolic syndrome risk factors that have been researched and identified as common in the population studied in the research article by Putz et al., "Integrated healthcare in a community-based mental health center: A longitudinal study of metabolic risk reduction," published in 2015 by the *Journal of Social Service Research*. A free abstract is available online (see Bibliography for details). Table 4.11 outlines, at a high level, the medical co-morbidities frequently encountered in a behavioral health population:

Table 4.11 Common Co-Morbid Conditions in the Behavioral Health Population, Especially Those with Serious Mental Illness (SMI)

Name of Condition	ICD-10-CM Chapter Location	Examples of Conditions
Obesity	Ch. 4, E66 codes	Overweight conditions contributing to behavioral health
Smoking, Respiratory	Ch. 5, F17, J40–J47	Chronic obstructive pulmonary disease, emphysema, asthma
Diabetes Mellitus	Ch. 4, E08–E13	Type 1, Type 2, controlled, uncontrolled
Cardiovascular	Ch.9, I-codes	Essential hypertension, coronary artery disease, high cholesterol

Other Conditions That You May Encounter in Practice

Additional code categories that may be helpful to clinicians are listed in Table 4.12. If you treat a certain population of behavioral health clients who have similar profiles, or if there is a higher incidence of certain medical conditions in the population you treat, then going through the ICD-10-CM Tabular Index to identify these codes, and their corresponding levels of specificity, is a critical step.

While it may seem cumbersome to go through all 21 Chapters of the ICD-10-CM codes and identify categories that are the most frequently-used subset seen at your place of practice, it is enormously imperative for clinical accuracy. The clinical imperative here is to actually assign a diagnosis code to the current situation, not merely notate it in the text or narrative portion of the medical record. The specificity and detailed nature of the ICD-10-CM enable us to code and track conditions for epidemiology and research purposes. Utilization of accurate and thorough coding and diagnosing is a benefit to all. By using HIT and data analysis, we can derive a tremendous amount of helpful information for improving population health.

Table 4.12 Other Useful ICD-10-CM Codes for Behavioral Health

Code Number Block*	ICD-10 Description/Examples
R10–R13	Abdominal and pelvic pain; nausea and vomiting; aphagia and dysphagia
R30–R39	Symptoms and signs involving the genitourinary system: incontinence
R41	Other symptoms and signs involving cognitive functions and awareness: amnesias, cognitive decline
R45	Symptoms and signs involving emotional state: hostility, anhedonia, **suicidal and homicidal ideations**
R46	Symptoms and signs involving appearance and behavior: very low level of personal hygiene, slowness and poor responsiveness
R47–R49	Symptoms and signs involving speech and voice: aphasia, dyslexia, apraxia
R63	Symptoms and signs concerning food and fluid intake: polydipsia, underweight
T39–T50	Poisoning by, adverse effects of, and underdosing of drugs, medicaments and biological substances; poisoning by aspirin/ heroin, opioids, etc. intentional self-harm
T58	Toxic effect of carbon monoxide
T71	Asphyxiations
X71–X83	Intentional self-harm: intentional self-harm by sharp object, jumping/lying in front of a motor vehicle
X92–Y08	Assault: behaviors directed towards others such as by handgun, drowning, blunt objects
Y07	Perpetrator of assault, maltreatment, and neglect
Z03.89	Encounter for observation for suspected diseases and conditions ruled out: this code is frequently used by State Medicaid agencies, children's services who require a diagnosis code but in which there is NO diagnosis.

*For specific code numbers, please refer to the ICD-10-CM Tabular Index.

Summary

In closing, this chapter discusses the various methods for conceptualizing and assigning diagnoses in the behavioral health clinical setting. Specifically, we have looked at the differences in language and clinical criteria between the DSM-5 and the ICD-10 Clinical Descriptions and Diagnostic Guidelines (CDDG). Some further considerations include:

1. Given the differences between the manuals, implementing a systematized approach to assigning diagnoses would be considered best practice.
2. It is imperative to ascertain how, when, and to what degree of specificity to assign medical diagnoses alongside mental health diagnoses.
3. Best practice is to diagnose and code for intentional self-harm (X-codes).
4. A clinical policy about the utilization practices of each manual and corresponding diagnostic criteria is recommended to promote consistency and clarity in a practice.
5. Having a clinical policy regarding the DSM and ICD is also helpful to aiding the goals of any Compliance Program.
6. When assigning a diagnosis to a client, it is important that the clinician understand the language differences, how diagnoses flow downstream to the payer and explain these concepts to the client.
7. The cornerstone of quality treatment, and ultimate success in clinical treatment, is to have a thorough and accurate diagnosis from which to derive the treatment plan and objectives.

Bibliography

American Psychiatric Association. (2013). *Diagnostic and Statistical Manual of Mental Disorders*, 5th edn. Washington, DC: American Psychiatric Association. Retrieved May 16, 2016 from http://dx.doi.org/10.1176/appi.books.9780890425596.

American Psychiatric Association. (2013). *DSM-5 Autism Spectrum Disorder Fact Sheet*. Retrieved April 1, 2016 from www.dsm5.org/Documents/Autism%20Spectrum%20Disorder%20Fact%20Sheet.pdf.

American Psychiatric Association. (2016). *DSM-5 Update: Supplement to Diagnostic and Statistical Manual of Mental Disorders*, 5th edn. Retrieved July 8, 2016 from http://dsm.psychiatryonline.org/pb-assets/dsm/update/DSM5Update2015.pdf.

Bhad, R., Lal, R., & Balhara, Y. P. S. (2015, October–November). Disorders related to use of psychoactive substances in DSM-5: Changes and challenges. *Indian Journal of Psychological Medicine, 37*(4), 470–2. Retrieved April 28, 2016 from www.ncbi.nlm.nih.gov/pmc/articles/PMC4676222/.

Cooper, J. E., & Sartorius, N. (2013). *A Companion to the Classification of Mental Disorders*. New York, NY: Oxford University Press.

De Hert, M., Correll, C. U., Bobes, J., Cetkovich-Bakmas, M., Cohen, D., Asai, I., . . . & Leucht, S. (2011). Physical illness in patients with severe mental disorders. I. Prevalence, impact of medications and disparities in health care. *World Psychiatry, 10*(1), 52–77. Retrieved April 28, 2016 from www.ncbi.nlm.nih.gov/pmc/articles/PMC3048500/.

First, M. B., Reed, G. M., Hyman, S. E., & Saxena, S. (2015, February 5). The development of the ICD-11 clinical descriptions and diagnostic guidelines for mental and behavioural disorders. *World Psychiatry, 14*(1), 82–90. Retrieved April 28, 2016 from www.ncbi.nlm.nih.gov/pmc/articles/PMC4329901/.

Frances, A. J., & Nardo, J. M. (2013). ICD-11 should not repeat the mistakes made by DSM-5. *The British Journal of Psychiatry, 203*(1), 1–2. DOI: 10.1192/bjp.bp.113.127647.

Hoffmann, N. G., & Kopak, A. M. (2015, April). How well do the DSM·5 alcohol use disorder designations map to the ICD·10 disorders? *Alcoholism: Clinical and Experimental Research, 39*(4), 697–701. DOI: 10.1111/acer.12685. Retrieved from www.ncbi.nlm.nih.gov/pubmed/25778707.

Norko, M. A., & Fitch, W. L. (2014). DSM-5 and substance use disorders: Clinicolegal implications. *Journal of the American Academy of Psychiatry and the Law Online, 42*(4), 443–52.

Putz, J. W., Sapir, H. E., Macy, J. T., Lieberman, T. E., Forster, S. E., Reece, M., . . . & Frasure, K. A. (2015). Integrated healthcare in a community-based mental health center: A longitudinal study of metabolic risk reduction. *Journal of Social Service Research, 41*(5), 584–93. Retrieved February 12, 2016 from www.tandfonline.com/doi/full/10.1080/01488376.2015.1072761.

Tandon, R., Gaebel, W., Barch, D. M., Bustillo, J., Gur, R. E., Heckers, S., . . . & Van Os, J. (2013). Definition and description of schizophrenia in the DSM-5. *Schizophrenia Research, 150*(1), 3–10. DOI: 10.1016/j.schres.2013.05.028.

World Health Organization. (1992). *The ICD-10 Classification of Mental and Behavioral Disorders: Diagnostic Criteria for Research*. 120–21, 292. Geneva: World Health Organization.

5 Understanding SNOMED CT

SNOMED CT stands for Systematized Nomenclature of Medicine, Clinical Terms. SNOMED CT is a standardized, "controlled" medical terminology that supports the capture of client health care information in an electronic health record (EHR) system. Information captured can later be retrieved and used for multiple purposes, or exchanged during transitions of care between multiple care specialties and sites of care. SNOMED CT reduces variability in the way clinical data are captured and encoded, thereby allowing information to be aggregated in a semantically meaningful way; aggregated data can ultimately contribute to improvements in care delivery. It might be helpful to picture SNOMED CT as the world's biggest thesaurus specifically designed for the healthcare field.

SNOMED CT is becoming an integral part of the healthcare industry worldwide as EHRs with the system built in become more widely adopted. Clinicians may already hear the term "SNOMED CT" referenced in practice settings, so having a basic understanding is essential. It is important that providers understand how SNOMED CT is utilized and will impact the behavioral health industry. It is not an easily graspable topic, but this chapter attempts to introduce and demonstrate the value of SNOMED CT to practitioners, researchers, and the science and technology industries.

SNOMED CT is a system of ontology: "a branch of metaphysics concerned with the nature and relations of being" (Merriam-Webster Dictionary, n.d.). It is a way of correlating related concepts to each other for purposes of easy retrieval from a computer system and for systemizing overall comprehension. Historically, with the lack of standardization of paper medical records, it has been difficult to effectively and comprehensively grasp and communicate the client's complete health condition. Now, with the utilization of EHRs, information is now grouped into select "data sets" and is specifically coded and defined, producing a more accurate clinical picture at client transfer and upon discharge.

Why is SNOMED CT important to behavioral health clinicians and systems? The current healthcare trends indicate that clients will no longer receive healthcare service delivery in segmented settings, such as private practices. Instead, integrated care models offering treatment across a wider continuum of care are being used. In order to achieve the overall goals of population health and patient safety, it is imperative that information being exchanged between care providers electronically is commonly understood. Think of SNOMED CT as similar to the CPT coding system: one CPT number represents a service delivery, with a standardized definition, and a common definition that is universally understood.

SNOMED CT is one of the standard code systems specified for use in EHRs and it supports the ability of information in disparate EHRs to be retrieved and electronically exchanged for purposes of client care. EHRs are also critical sources of data for health statistics, epidemiology, and research purposes, to name a few uses. Many varieties of EHRs exist, ranging from the very basic to the more elaborate, fully certified systems. Examples of how SNOMED CT is working within an EHR can be:

- maintain an up-to-date problem list of current and active diagnoses;
- record client family history as structured data;
- identify and report cancer cases to registries;
- record and chart changes in vital signs;
- record smoking status;
- automatically link problem lists (driven by SNOMED CT) to Medline or other educational resources that can be easily accessed and printed out for clients;
- provide a summary, or continuity-of-care, record for transitions of care.

By establishing a common language among all medical disciplines, SNOMED CT improves semantic interoperability and reinforces the idea that mental health and substance use conditions can be inextricably linked to the other health problems. In other words, there is a dire need to capture data in EHRs in a way that enhances the delivery of healthcare while enabling the same information used to document the delivery of care to be retrieved, aggregated, analyzed and exchanged at a later date.

SNOMED CT is maintained by the International Health Terminology Standards Organization (IHTSDO), a not-for-profit association that is owned and governed by its membership, based in Denmark. According to IHSTDO (2014, 6), SNOMED CT is:

> clinical information recorded using identifiers that refer to concepts that are formally defined as part of the terminology . . . [it] supports recording of clinical information at appropriate levels of detail using relevant clinical concepts . . . [it] allows information to be entered using synonyms suitable to local preferences while recording information consistently and comparably.

SNOMED CT is huge: it has more than 300,000 concepts, 779,000 descriptions, 19 hierarchies, and 1.5 million relationships. And, when we consider that it was intended to be embedded in electronic healthcare systems, it should be no surprise when the *SNOMED CT Technical Implementation Guide* is close to 757 pages long!

SNOMED CT: Its Development Over Time

The following itemization shows the history and development of SNOMED CT over time:

- 1965: The College of American Pathologists' (CAP) Systematized Nomenclature of Pathology (SNOP) was published.
- 1975: The College of American Pathologists expanded the itemization and called it Systematized Nomenclature of Medicine, SNOMED.
- 1979: SNOMED II was developed.
- 1980s: The UK's National Health Service developed Clinical Terms Version 3 (CTV3),
- 1993: SNOMED International, or SNOMED 3, was developed.
- 2000: The College of American Pathologists and Kaiser Permanente developed the logic-based SNOMED Reference Terminology (RT).
- 1998–2002: CTV3 and SNOMED RT were merged to produce the first version of SNOMED CT.
- 2007: SNOMED CT was acquired by the International Health Terminology Standards Organization (IHTSDO), based in Denmark.
- SNOMED CT is open source and free to use by anyone in a member country. This includes EHR software developers in member countries.

- The National Library of Medicine in the USA is an official member organization of IHTSDO.
- SNOMED CT, like the ICD, is an international standardized and controlled clinical vocabulary that provides clinicians with the clinical content necessary to document the provision of care, using terms that clinicians are familiar with and which provide standard meaning.

Starting with nine member countries in 2007, there are now more than 28 countries belonging to IHTSDO, and more join every year. The International Edition of SNOMED CT is licensed by IHTSDO, and updates to the list are distributed every July and January. SNOMED CT can be used under a free license by member countries, or purchased. It is also used in more than 40 non-member countries for low-cost licenses. The tab-delimited release files include versioning data that allows changes to be tracked over time and supports generational views of earlier releases. This historical reference is helpful should a clinician need to access older versions. At this juncture in healthcare history, it is important to remember that SNOMED CT is a work in progress, always developing and improving; IHTSDO welcomes input and feedback about SNOMED CT from any interested party.

SNOMED CT is published in a variety of languages, and member countries can customize it to fit their unique needs. It is designed to support the national "extensions" (i.e. country-specific variations) that enable the addition of local translations and/or dialect variants, without undermining the global representation of meanings. This protocol is similar to the USA adapting the ICD-10 to produce the ICD-10-CM, which is unique to the USA. While SNOMED CT has country-specific editions, all editions are built on top of the international edition. It is the use of the descriptions and "RefSets" (discussed later in this chapter) that allows for country and language-specific editions.

SNOMED CT is different than a diagnostic classification system such as the ICD or the DSM because it is a *controlled medical terminology* built according to defining principles. It contains the broad range of concepts required to be fully expressive in an EHR. In fact, the DSM is simply just a *diagnostic manual* available for arriving at a clinical diagnosis. The ICD is a *coding system, with corresponding clinical descriptions and diagnostic guidelines* to support the assignment of the ICD-10 diagnostic codes. Keep in mind that the codes in the DSM are actually repurposed ICD codes and the DSM is not a code system itself. The ICD is open source and free, engaging the worldwide community in contributing to the development of the series. Like the ICD-10, SNOMED CT is also open source and open to improvements and suggestions by the community at large. It would make sense to eliminate extraneous systems that confuse providers, clinicians, third parties, and even state and local governments.

How SNOMED CT Works: Structure and Components

SNOMED CT is massive and encompasses terms covering clinical medicine and the veterinary sciences. It is *a controlled medical terminology* that gives providers a real opportunity to make the clinical medical record meaningful, especially EHRs. Its concepts are based on formal logic-based definitions that communicate their meaning. As behavioral health clinicians, only small subsets of the SNOMED CT terms may be applicable to our day-to-day work. Yet the concepts and terms are drawn from the same vocabulary that other care providers will be using, and they can facilitate a more seamless, semantically accurate view of the client's condition.

You can search SNOMED CT by accessing the content through a number of "browser" applications found on the IHTSDO homepage. In this context, the term "browser" is used as a specific type of search engine on the IHSDTO's website, and does not reference how one accesses the Internet (e.g. Internet Explorer, Mozilla, etc.). One of the most efficient ways of understanding SNOMED CT is to go into a browser and conduct a search for a certain term. Look at the search results and begin to comprehend the relationships between the terms found in the search. You may also want to note how the concept has been defined in relationship to its hierarchies and relationship details.

Hands-on experience with a browser is very valuable and will ultimately help the clinician understand how SNOMED CT is constructed and developed. Care should be taken in choosing a browser because browsers are country-specific. It will be important to pull up the browser that corresponds to your country's SNOMED CT Extension. If you are in the USA, you will want to make sure you are looking at the US edition browser of the IHSTDO's SNOMED CT.

Next, since SNOMED CT is concept-based, it is important to understand the relationship between terms and identifiers. The scope of the system is broad, meaning that it includes concepts representing a myriad of information that needs to be recorded in clinical records. As a result, practitioners from different disciplines and specialties can use SNOMED CT to record appropriate data at different stages in the delivery of care. This standardization leads to better coordination, continuity, integration of care and, ultimately, improved population health.

For the purposes of this textbook, only the key concepts of SNOMED CT that clinicians may encounter will be discussed. SNOMED CT has evolved to help computer systems process encoded healthcare information recorded at the point of care, whenever that information is needed. This facilitates information that is sent between disparate EHRs, whether it is a database query for reporting purposes, or for analytical purposes.

The way SNOMED CT is designed and implemented may be more comprehensible to those in the computer sciences (or in the philosophy industry) than in the behavioral health sciences. It is hoped that the utility of SNOMED CT will be understood by the community of providers, who can ultimately contribute to future editions if gaps are discovered in the terminology.

Concepts

SNOMED CT concepts represent the embodiment of a particular meaning of clinical thoughts, ranging from very general expressions to very specific descriptions. Every concept represents a unique clinical meaning, described by using "terms." Terms, in SNOMED CT, are character strings that consist of words, phrases, and human-readable representations that convey meaning. Each concept is referenced by a unique, numeric, and machine-readable SNOMED CT identifier code number (SCTID) that does not have any ascribed human-interpretable meaning.

SNOMED CT concepts are arranged in hierarchies and are related to one another by relationships. The relationships between the concepts provide computer-readable definitions for each concept, which allows for consistent retrieval of clinical information from EHRs for purposes of treatment, reporting, research, and other analyses. The hierarchies are related to one another by "is-a" relationships (see below), and have several subcategories branching out from them. In other words, SNOMED CT is poly-hierarchical and concepts may fall under several related categories. The other items related to concepts (parents, parent-child, subtypes, and supertypes) are beyond the scope of this textbook.

The Fully Specified Name (FSN) for the top level SNOMED CT concept (also called the "root concept"), is SNOMED CT Concept (SNOMED RT+CTV3). The SCTID is 138875005. Under the root concept are general concepts referred to as "top-level concepts." Most of the clinically relevant concepts in SNOMED CT fall under one of the following 17 top-level concepts:

1. Clinical finding
2. Physical object
3. Procedure

4. Physical force
5. Situation with explicit context
6. Event
7. Observable entity
8. Environments and geographical locations
9. Body structure
10. Social context
11. Organism
12. Staging and scales
13. Substance
14. Qualifier value
15. Pharmaceutical/biological product
16. Record artifact
17. Specimen.

Not surprisingly, while there are many concepts in SNOMED CT, it is most likely that only a small subset applicable to your specialty area may have been embedded into the EHR (i.e. are already in the system/EHR and ready to go). A good question to ask your EHR vendor partner is to what extent is SNOMED CT used in your application. You may not visually recognize when you encounter SNOMED CT in the EHR. For some EHR systems, the unique identifier will be prefaced by "SCT," which represents the SNOMED CT code.

Descriptions

A description is a narrative set of textual descriptors assigned to every concept, intended to represent the way that a concept is commonly referenced in practice. Descriptions provide the human readable form of a concept. In other words, descriptions are words we can read as opposed to computer code, numbers, or logic.

When one clinician uses a term, such as "depression," it can have very different meanings for different clinicians. How can we effectively communicate, for purposes of continuity and transfers of care, what is the client's health status? This is where SNOMED CT becomes invaluable, and complementary, to the ICD series. That said, SNOMED CT is similar to, but different from, the ICD series. Keep in mind that the ICD is a classification system, whereas SNOMED CT is a reference terminology system.

Another way of explaining SNOMED CT is to recall how there are many different ways to describe one clinical condition, procedure, or situation. For example, different specialty providers from internal medicine, social work, or psychiatry, working with the same client, will each have their own clinical terminology to describe the same state of depression. Some may use the word "depression" whereas others may use the term "depressive state" or even "depressive disorder." There can be many ways to describe a single concept but in the integrated healthcare service delivery model, it is imperative that we have a common language across disciplines that we can trace back to a single, standardized meaning. With SNOMED CT, every term, phrase, or concept is connected to a single, standardized concept.

The multiple descriptions of a single, unique concept is what gives SNOMED CT its "thesaurus" feature. An example, using Generalized Anxiety Disorder (taken from the US Edition 20160301), is illustrated in Table 5.1:

Table 5.1 Term Example of SNOMED CT Description for Generalized Anxiety Disorder

Concept ID (aka SCTID)		Description Term	Acceptability	Description ID	Notes/ Commentary by Textbook Authors
21897009	F	Generalized anxiety disorder (disorder)	Preferred	751243014	The Concept ID 21897009 is uniquely associated with the concept of the diagnosis Generalized Anxiety Disorder. F = Fully Specified Name (FSN); S = Synonyms: Are terms used for display in the EHR or to select and search for concepts. Each concept may have one or more synonyms, and this allows users to use terms they prefer when referring to a specific clinical concept. Term: This indicates whether the Description Term is the Fully Specified Name or a synonym associated with with unique concept identifier.
	S	Generalized anxiety disorder	Preferred	36731013	
	S	GAD – Generalized anxiety disorder	Acceptable	481155011	

Table 5.1 *continued*

Concept ID (aka SCTID)	Description Term	Acceptability	Description ID	Notes/ Commentary by Textbook Authors
				Acceptability: This indicates the preferred or accepted descriptions for a concept. Of the Synonyms listed in the Description Term column, they will be labeled as preferred or acceptable.
				Description ID: Each description is also associated with its own identifier. These unique identifiers are used internally by SNOMED CT to link human readable terms to concepts.

Table 5.1 gives you a visual representation of the different clinical words or phrases that have been determined to possess the same meaning and associated with a single unique concept.

Relationships

SNOMED CT Relationships associate or link between two concepts together. Within SNOMED CT, there are four types of relationship. Each type is assigned to different SNOMED CT concepts: Defining, Qualifying, Historical, and Additional. It is the Defining relationships that are used to model SNOMED CT concepts and that create the logical definitions that allow concepts to be processed by computers. However, not all hierarchies in SNOMED CT have defining attributes. The highest priority was given to developing defining attributes that would be useful for aggregated analysis of outcomes, decision support, and knowledge-based practice guidelines in a clinical setting. As a result, defining attributes were first assigned to hierarchies where retrieval of clinical data is most useful and relevant: Procedure, Clinical Finding, Event, Situation with Explicit Context, Pharmaceutical/Biological Product, Physical Object and Specimen.

An attribute relationship is an association between two concepts that specifies a defining characteristic of one of the concepts. Each attribute relationship has a name (i.e. the type of relationship) and a value (i.e. the destination of the relationship). For example, the combination of the attribute relationships and "is-a" relationships associated with a concept represent the logical definition of that concept. The logical concept definition includes one or more supertypes (represented by "is-a" relationships), and a set of defining attributes that differentiate it from any other concept definition.

Each defining attribute relationship represents a characteristic of a SNOMED CT concept. SNOMED CT currently uses more than 50 defining attributes. The set of rules that define the types of relationships permitted between concepts is referred to as the "SNOMED CT Concept Model." It is the Concept Model that specifies the set of concepts to which an attribute can be applied and the permitted set of values for each attribute.

RefSets

Finally, you may hear the term "RefSets" which stands for Reference Sets. RefSets are specialized types of SNOMED CT files that allow the terminology to be customized for a particular country, organization, specialty or local situation. For example, RefSets can be used to constrain what it makes sense to record in the EHR and what information is allowed to be exchanged under certain circumstances. In addition, RefSets can used to provide a map between SNOMED CT concepts and other code system terminologies such as ICD-10-CM and LOINC (Logical Observation Identifiers Names and Codes).

SNOMED CT in the EHR

In addition to SNOMED CT being a standardized terminology, it affords providers the opportunity to make the clinical medical record meaningful. Keep in mind that SNOMED CT is a controlled clinical vocabulary designed for computer systems to collect, connect, aggregate, exchange, and translate health information for multiple purposes.

Where will a behavioral health clinician most likely interact with SNOMED CT in the EHR? In many EHR systems or medical records, there is an item called "patient problem list" or "POV" ("purpose of visit"). Other terms used for this may be "presenting problem" or "chief complaint." This is an item that is typically found at the beginning of the medical record that has a running list of the client's active, ongoing, and/or chronic problems. This list is usually updated at every healthcare encounter for efficacy. Behavioral health clinicians will likely interact with SNOMED CT when recording diagnoses and other clinical findings.

CMS defines "problem list" for purposes of the Meaningful Use EHR Incentive Program as *"a list of current and active diagnoses as well as past diagnoses relevant to the current care of the patient."* With this rationale, clinical terminology standardization becomes evident and supports the objectives of true exchange of electronic information and semantic interoperability.

Another way in which SNOMED CT impacts the clinician is through the functionality of clinical decision support (CDS) rules. CDS rules are a series of logic-based formulas established to alert the clinician when certain conditions are met, or need attention. For example, a CDS rule could be set up that prompts the clinician to perform a suicide risk assessment if "suicidal ideation" is itemized in the problem list. The clinician can then make a decision to conduct the assessment or dismiss it.

SNOMED CT may be used to automatically link client educational information sheets to problem lists for easy retrieval and printing purposes. In this way, the end user does not have to open another screen, browser, or link, to search and find educational materials. This automation can promote point-of-care efficiency.

SNOMED CT terms are also used in other sections of the EHR: family history, smoking status, allergy and drug reactions. In other words, SNOMED CT is a language that is likely to be used throughout the medical record, but specifically at certain critical data-capture points in order to gather concrete information about health conditions, situations, and provide consistent collaborative care to our clients across multiple provider specialties or care settings. Certainly, this will enable us to provide a standardized database of clinical terminology for health statistics and epidemiology purposes.

While massive and comprehensive, one can begin to appreciate how SNOMED CT fits into many segments of the behavioral healthcare industry. From EHRs to integrated care service delivery models, evidence-based practices and clinical decision support rules embedded in the EHR, SNOMED CT is the common denominator that ties healthcare information technology and exchange together. For example, Transitions of Care (TOC) or Continuity of Care Documents (CCDs), and/or electronic summaries about a client's care at your organization that are sent to another organization, will contain SNOMED CT terminology and concepts. SNOMED CT will also display on diagnosis pages in the EHR, and in client portals to help describe the conditions for which the client was treated. There may be ICD codes and diagnoses listed as well, but the standardized data elements reinforce the expectation that a client's "problem history" will be conveyed using SNOMED CT terminology.

SNOMED CT's biggest function in the information system is to consistently, comprehensively, and reliably represent clinically relevant information and data. It is a way for clinicians to standardize the documentation and description of how we implement and deliver healthcare services across health disciplines, state lines, and the globe. It gives us a comprehensive system of clinically-relevant terms, descriptors, and clinical names that are grouped a certain way to describe a single condition, such as depression or headache.

SNOMED CT plays a critical role in health information exchange because it enables automation within healthcare information systems, and standardizes the meaning of healthcare concepts across the world. It also provides different specialty clinicians with a common language to describe a single client's condition, enabling greater continuity of care.

Importance and Implications of SNOMED CT

Why is SNOMED CT important and how does it benefit integrated care delivery models? The answer to this question was put forth in one sentence in the IHTSDO *SNOMED CT Starter Guide* (2014, 6):

> The objective of IHTSDO and all users of SNOMED CT is to facilitate the accurate recording and sharing of clinical and related health information and the semantic interoperability of health records.

SNOMED CT clinical terms are, behind the scenes, mapped to functionality in your EHR like the ICD codes. Clinical decision support rules are also hard-coded, tabled, and mapped. The use of SNOMED CT gives a clinician, regardless of area of specialty or country, a standardized way to represent clinical conditions and phrases. SNOMED CT is a controlled vocabulary, meaning that terms are clinically validated and have the same meaning regardless of who is using the term or in which country they reside. In other words, SNOMED CT is a clinical terminology with *a global scope covering a wide range of disciplines and requirements, a common language to all of healthcare.*

As a result of its broad scope, one of the benefits of SNOMED CT is a reduction of healthcare disciplinary boundary effects that arise from the use of different terminologies or coding systems by different clinicians, departments, or countries. In other words, the family physician, internist, radiologist, and behavioral health clinicians can all "speak" the same language. This standardization allows for comprehensive sharing and reuse of structured clinical information and plays a critical role in integrated service delivery of healthcare. Another benefit of SNOMED CT is that the same data can be processed and presented in ways that serve different purposes.

The data that is contained in an information system, specifically an EHR, is a goldmine for research. By having SNOMED CT as a part of the EHR system, we can leverage data analytics by creating queries to find commonalities, patterns, incidence, and causes of certain health conditions. Genomic and metabolic research can be conducted to help understand the underpinnings of mental illness across the globe. More importantly, the use of SNOMED CT brings behavioral health clinicians into alignment with other healthcare disciplines.

One of the biggest shifts behavioral health clinicians will need to make is moving away from the DSM language to the universal, global terminology, nomenclature, and language. While good-faith efforts are being made to map DSM-5 codes to SNOMED CT terms and codes, this transition or "crosswalk" is not seamless. Therefore, we encounter the same challenges with SNOMED CT that we have with the different diagnostic classification systems, DSM and ICD: they are disparate systems that may create confusion and misalignment in the industry. Having a globally agreed-upon standardized system would certainly offer world health experts significant advantages, and ultimately provide relief to clinicians who have historically needed to juggle multiple systems.

With the release of ICD-11, the new ICD-11 CDDGs, and SNOMED CT, behavioral health clinicians worldwide will have the most current and open-source/free reference set of materials available. One of the key issues is for regulatory third-party entities using a universal straightforward, integrated system. In the USA, medical policies and reimbursements will fully and solely be tied to the ICD and SNOMED CT series, thus eliminating out-of-date diagnostic and record-keeping protocols. It will be a very exciting time for the worldwide behavioral health industry when the ICD-11, ICD-11 CDDG, and SNOMED CT converge.

Summary

Behavioral healthcare clinicians are unknowingly likely to interact with SNOMED CT in their health information technology system or EHR. Having a standardized, unified meaning assigned to a term or concept is important for a variety of reasons and it is anticipated that SNOMED CT will become increasingly more important to healthcare delivery models in the years ahead.

Many Systems, Confusion, and a Brief Summary:

SNOMED CT Terms

A scientifically-validated, standardized language used in EHRs across disciplines for purposes of improving interoperability and decreasing disparities in systems across international healthcare.

ICD Codes

Code numbers, representative of the clinical diagnosis or condition treated in the healthcare encounter. In the USA, also used for billing and reimbursement purposes.

DSM series

Diagnostic manuals that contain behavioral health clinical descriptions and the diagnostic criteria to help guide the clinician in arriving at a diagnosis.

The ICD's Clinical Descriptions and Diagnostic Guidelines

The ICD's companion diagnostic manual with associated descriptions of a diagnostic condition related to a specific ICD-10 diagnosis code.

Bibliography

Bowman, S. E. (2005, May 25). *Coordination of SNOMED CT and ICD-10: Getting the Most Out of Electronic Health Record Systems*. Retrieved May 13, 2016 from http://library.ahima.org/doc?oid=106578#.VzZB2PkrKUk.

Centers for Medicare & Medicaid Services. (2014, May). *Eligible Professional Meaningful Use Core Measures, Measure 3 of 13: Stage 1, 2014 Definition*. Retrieved April 2, 2016 from www.cms.gov/Regulations-and-Guidance/Legislation/EHRIncentivePrograms/downloads/3_Maintain_Problem_ListEP.pdf.

Healthit.gov. (2016, March 3). *Certified Health IT Product List (CHPL)*. Retrieved May 13, 2016 from www.healthit.gov/policy-researchers-implementers/certified-health-it-product-list-chpl.

International Health Terminology Standards Development Organization. (1999). *SNOMED CT Systematized Nomenclature of Medicine, Clinical Terms*. Retrieved April 1, 2016 from www.ihtsdo.org/snomed-ct/.

International Health Terminology Standards Development Organization. (2014, February). *SNOMED CT Starter Guide*. Retrieved April 2, 2016 from http://ihtsdo.org/fileadmin/user_upload/doc/download/doc_StarterGuide_Current-en-US_INT_20140222.pdf.
International Health Terminology Standards Development Organization. (2015, January). *SNOMED CT Technical Implementation Guide: January 2015 International Release (US English)*. Retrieved April 2, 2016 from http://ihtsdo.org/fileadmin/user_upload/doc/download/doc_TechnicalImplementationGuide_Current-en-US_INT_20150131.pdf.
Merriam-Webster Dictionary. (n.d.). *Ontology* [Def. 1]. Retrieved November 11, 2016 from www.merriam-webster.com/dictionary/ontology.

6 Coding and Documentation Compliance in Behavioral Health

This chapter addresses ICD-10-CM compliance, coding and documentation requirements for best practice. It is written from the vantage point of helping students prepare for workforce compliance in coding and documentation. Curriculums teach clinical process and content to students, and internships/practicums help operationalize the material they have learned. However, students are sometimes very surprised to learn upon entering the workforce that there are regulatory and business processes that govern their day-to-day tasks. Administrators of facilities spend a lot of resources onboarding new staff; therefore, part of this chapter's objective is to help you prepare your students for tomorrow's workforce. For schools looking to increase their enrollment rates, preparing students with workforce readiness knowledge and skills is both advantageous and critical.

SAMSHA and HRSA provide clear and comprehensive expectations that readiness of tomorrow's behavioral health workforce will involve the core competencies to support healthcare reform initiatives and improve population health. One of these core competencies is integrated care models, which incorporate our clients' medical issues into the behavioral health record and treatment. In order for this to be accomplished, the behavioral health industry needs to come into alignment with the medical industry in regard to documentation, data collection, practices, and standardized processes. This chapter will illuminate these considerations as we move forward to improve population and world health.

Coding and documenting are not routinely taught in our medical schools, nor in behavioral health graduate programs. Yet, so much wasted time, resources, and efforts could be minimized if curriculums began to weave coding and documentation into their curriculums, even in an abbreviated manner. Unfortunately, most clinicians learn the hard way: peer review, supervision, coding department queries, and challenging chart audits. It is far more effective and preventive to teach good coding and documentation protocol in the classroom than it is to have to rectify errors in the practice world.

Clinical Practice Considerations

This section will specifically address these behavioral health clinical documentation areas:

- documentation for services rendered and diagnosis assigned
- coding correctly for billing and reimbursement.

One of the most comprehensive compilations of compliance and documentation in the behavioral health industry comes from a book published by the America Health Information Management Association (AHIMA), titled *Documentation and Reimbursement for Behavioral Healthcare Services,* written in 2005. While AHIMA is considered an industry leader in the medical arena, it has also been active in behavioral health sectors for quite some time. Many of the third-party payer requirements for coding and documenting behavioral health services likely comes from AHIMA's suggestions, guidelines, policies, input, and standards, including accrediting bodies like the Joint Commission and Council on Accreditation.

ICD Documentation Requirements for Services and Diagnoses

Most states in the USA, as well as the US federal government, set forth laws and statutes that dictate what needs to be included in a legal medical record, or in the case of HIPAA, a Designated Record Set (DRS). A client's behavioral health record typically will consist of both administrative and clinical information. Broadly speaking and for purposes of this chapter, administrative information in the record is considered to be items such as demographic information, family contacts, third-party involvements, consents, Release of

Information data, and other items. Clinical documentation includes items such as the diagnoses, assessments, medications, treatment plans and goals, session notes, psychological testing, interventions, and client's participation in treatment.

If you are not familiar with your state's definition of what legally constitutes a medical record, it is imperative that each provider has comprehensive knowledge of the mandates set forth by their regulating entities, such as HIPAA, accrediting agencies, specific contracts with third parties, regulatory bodies and even the state's Medicaid office.

In fact, CMS issued a document in December 2015 entitled "Medicaid Documentation for Behavioral Health Practitioners." According to this document, regarding documented services, reimbursable behavioral health services must:

- meet each state's Medicaid program participation rules;
- reflect medical necessity and levels of care as defined by the state to justify the treatment and clinical rationale for medically necessary treatment;
- reflect active treatment provided;
- be complete, concise, accurate, and include face time;
- be legible, signed, dated, and available for review;
- be coded correctly for billing purposes.

It is this last item—*be coded correctly for billing purposes*—which clinicians need to follow strictly. When charting, each clinician will need to both justify the documented service for medical necessity as well as document that the treatment provided is congruent with the assessment, diagnosis, and treatment plan provided for that client. In addition to substantiating the diagnosis and justifying the type of service rendered, the duration and level of services should include documentation that, at a minimum, contains the following items:

1. clinical observations
2. interventions performed
3. client's response to the interventions.

"Be coded correctly for billing purposes," means that the ICD-10 CM coding and documentations standards are being followed (as discussed in Chapter 2) and that the diagnosis is substantiated to the highest degree of specificity known for that particular healthcare encounter. It also means that the ICD-10-CM codes are used and verified prior to submission on a healthcare claim and that these codes have come from the true, authenticated source: the ICD-10-CM

Tabular Index (as recommended by this textbook since most clinicians are not CPCs). A sample of documentation requirements for some diagnoses is included in the Appendix.

To achieve a high degree of compliance with coding and documentation standards, the documentation must: support the services that were provided and billed, be medically necessary, meet payers and regulatory requirements, support the diagnosis and treatment plan, and demonstrate the Golden Thread discussed earlier. Documentation of utilizing Evidence-Based Practices (EBPs) is critical for certain certifications or other requirements, both at an agency level, as well as at the clinical level. If these protocols are not followed, standardization will not be achieved and behavioral health clinicians will continue to document in ways that put the client, provider, and healthcare industry at risk.

In addition, it is critical to internal auditing programs to use audit tools based on the regulations, laws, EBP and standards, and the action of client care when looking for gaps in processes that can be improved upon by the clinician. Using EBPs and other scientifically-sound intervention steps then can be quantified and captured as data elements. This will then facilitate the collection of metrics for a variety of reporting and quality program initiatives.

Class Discussion:

CMS on Fidelity to ICD-10-CM Compliance

What Would You Do?

In the early 2016, CMS-Medicare began to deny claims for two diagnoses contained in the DSM-5 manual. Those diagnoses were: F20.9, Schizophrenia Unspecified and F43.10, Post-Traumatic Stress Disorder, Unspecified. These are the only two diagnostic codes in the DSM-5 listed for these disorders. In addition to causing significant revenue disruption, this action left a lot of clinicians wondering why the codes they used from the DSM-5 were being denied. The National Council on Behavioral Health, working with the American Psychiatric Association, began to gather some of the denied claims for purposes of trying to remedy the situation.

These two diagnoses are legitimate diagnosis codes in ICD-10-CM, and are the only ones itemized in the DSM-5, so it is easy to see how a clinician would be mistaken if they only used the DSM-5 as their reference. However, these codes do *not* meet the threshold for a specific diagnosis, such as the other types of Schizophrenia or Acute versus Chronic PTSD in the ICD-10-CM. From your reading of this book, the action taken by CMS would be seemingly correct if the client truly meets the coding and documentation criteria required for an "Unspecified" diagnosis (see Chapter 2). It is reasonable and understandable how CMS arrived at this decision since all HIPAA-covered entities (HIPAA-CEs) are mandated to use the ICD-10-CM system.

But how is anyone to know whether or not the client meets the Unspecified criteria? *Only a physical chart review or audit of the documentation would reveal this.* Audits are time consuming and very stressful. Can a payer set up their computer systems to kick back any Unspecified claims? Yes, they can, and the burden is on the clinician to have justified their utilization of an Unspecified diagnosis in the medical record at the point of care. Can you appeal this decision? Yes, but again this consumes resources. What if you know for a fact, and have documented, that your client of ten years is a Paranoid Schizophrenic but you submit F20.9, Schizophrenia, Unspecified because that is the only available code in your EHR system that only uses the digital DSM-5 version?

What happens if the EHR software vendor you use has loaded only the DSM-5 codes into the system, not the ICD-10-CM codes or Tabular Index, and you do not have access to the other specific Schizophrenia diagnoses that CMS is looking for, or PSTD-codes for acute and chronic? What about the X-codes, medical codes, and all the other possible codes?

Most vendors include a "hold harmless" (indemnity) clause in their contracts. Also contained in the contracts is a clause that the vendors will follow state and federal laws, of which using the ICD-10-CM codes is a law. Who is liable? Is this in violation of the federal law? If yes, then who is violating the law? Who pays the price? The provider organization, the EHR vendor, the clinician, and the client are all affected. It would be much simpler to have one standardized classification system for diagnosing and coding.

Finally, how would you "code correctly for billing purposes" and what process would you follow?

While every state or agency may decide to define the contents of a medical record differently, section 42 CFR 482.24 of the federal regulation code (i.e the "Conditions of Participation" for the Centers for Medicare and Medicaid Services) also defines what constitutes a "complete medical record." The CMS Manual System reiterates this definition in its guidance to clinicians. The key item to focus on is the word, "*complete.*" CMS defines "complete" in this way:

> All entries in the medical record must be complete. A medical record is considered complete if it contains sufficient information to identify the patient; *support the diagnosis/condition*; justify the care, treatment, and services; document the course and results of care, treatment, and services; *and promote continuity of care among providers*.
>
> (Centers for Medicare & Medicaid Services, 2012)

The two phrases, "support the diagnosis/condition" and "promote continuity of care among providers," are critical for demonstrating fidelity to the ICD-10-CM requirements and guidelines. With the emphasis of these requirements combined with the added level of specificity in the ICD-10-CM, the threshold for quality documentation in the behavioral health industry has been elevated to a level not seen before in the industry.

How does a clinician justify the diagnosis assigned to their client? Generally speaking, clinicians will need to:

- add details in the record to support the more specific ICD-10 diagnosis;
- link symptoms, complications and the manifestations to the diagnosis;
- understand that the diagnostic details needed will depend on the diagnosis and criteria.

A good way to think of this process is: "What would a Certified Coder or an Auditor do or look for in the record?" Certainly, the elements of accuracy, detail, specificity, and thoroughness are imperative. If clinical documentation does not support the diagnosis, then it becomes cloudy as to how the clinician arrived at such a diagnosis. In other words, the assigned diagnosis (that appears on the claim forms or to outside entities) *must* be based directly on the provider's documentation.

In compliance circles, the following saying is sometimes heard: "If it was not written, it was not done." For behavioral health clinicians, there is an inherent tension between documenting to meet all the regulatory requirements and medical necessity versus protecting a client's privacy and confidentiality. By supporting the diagnosis and condition, we are simply itemizing the intensity, frequency, and duration of the signs and symptoms our client is exhibiting. In other words, we need *solid clinical* documentation, not necessarily *more* documentation or verbiage in the medical record.

Below are some documentation strategies for supporting the diagnosis or condition assigned to your client through their treatment episode:

- Use a single diagnostic and coding classification system to extract your rationale for assigning a particular diagnosis.
- Choose to utilize the DSM-5, the ICD CDDGs, or a hybrid approach, making sure that your methodology is standardized, consistent, and itemized in a clinical policy.
- Itemize each of the signs, symptoms, frequency, intensity, and duration of the symptoms to justify the severity of the diagnosis given.
- Detail the degree of the client's challenges and how they are coping with the condition.
- Label, define, and discuss severity throughout the record at every opportunity.
- Document the level of impairment due to the condition or how the client will not progress developmentally due to the condition.
- List behaviors and motor symptoms, their duration, frequency, and intensity.
- Identify the client's level of functioning.
- Give a clinical rationale as to why this level of intervention is indicated at this time.
- Itemize clinical indicators (symptoms and severity) by history and within the last five days.
- Document any previous admissions.
- Document intent: accidental, intentional, undetermined, or intentional self-harm.
- Document using phrases or terms such as: acute versus chronic, with or without complications, with or without behavioral disturbance, with or without psychotic features, continuous versus episodic. Make this a regular habit.

The last topic to cover in this section on ICD documentation requirements involves the inclusion and clinical documentation of additional diagnoses that are the subject of clinical attention, or which impact the client's presentation. Specifically, some suggestions for improved documentation elements per diagnostic category are outlined in Table 6.1. This list is not exhaustive, and it will also be contingent on your practice's clinical policies and procedures.

Table 6.1 Clinical Area and Correlated Documentation Elements

Diagnostic Area	Documentation Suggestions by Authors
Medical	Have a clinical policy and procedure in place to determine specificity, number of character/digits coded. The list below is suggested by AHIMA, and may or may not apply to your practice:
	Disease type
	Disease acuity (mild, moderate, severe)
	Disease stage (acute, chronic, intermittent, recurrent, persistent, transient, major, most recent episode)
	Site specificity (arms, legs, etc.)
	Laterality (self-harm)
	Encounter type (initial, subsequent, sequela)
	Current condition vs. past history
	Relationship of condition to procedure (or intervention)
	Etiology
	Symptoms/manifestations associated with disease process
	External cause
Self-Harm	Site specificity, laterality, means, align chart note with diagnosis (e.g. sharp vs. blunt object)
Psychological	Intensity, duration, frequency, severity, scope of signs, symptoms, behaviors and manifestations

Class Discussion

Documentation Examples and Considerations

Look at the following two samples and discuss the strengths and challenges to each one.

1

You work in an outpatient substance use program and you write: "Client showed for her appointment. She was high on drugs. It was hard to have a session with her because of this but she did talk about the conflict with her boss." You then assign her the ICD-10-CM diagnosis of F14.151: Cocaine abuse with cocaine-induced psychotic disorder with hallucinations.

- How would you change the note to support the diagnosis you chose in the EHR and submitted to the third party?
- What elements would you add, or eliminate?

2

Betty Boo is a long-time client of the agency, 15 years to be exact. Almost every clinician has interacted with her over time. She always comes into her appointments looking and talking like Eeyore, from the Winnie-the-Pooh series. She also wears a red hat, purple shoes, and bright red lipstick smeared all over her face. You are a recently- graduated clinician, new to the agency. You see her for one session and after she leaves, you run into your colleague's office to discuss Betty Boo. You find out Betty Boo has been around for a very long time and everyone at your agency knows her. As a result of this information, you then assign her a diagnosis of Dysthymia and Histrionic Personality Disorder and justify this by indicating: "*Client is known to this agency.*" No itemization of symptoms, duration, frequency is given.

- What documentation issue(s) might be problematic in this chart note?
- How might you change the chart note to substantiate the diagnosis?

The above samples were extracted from actual medical records in 2014, with details changed, of course, to disguise identifying information.

Considerations:

1. How often do you perform a full diagnostic assessment and/or update the diagnosis?
2. How do you support the ongoing treatment of a diagnosis and reflect that the diagnosis is still active in the ongoing session/chart notes?
3. How would you document, on a continual basis, for a client who has four diagnoses, including medical diagnoses?
4. Everyone at your organization has a different opinion for updating and substantiating diagnoses. How might a clinical policy and procedure help?

How would you write the chart/session notes for the two samples above?

Clinical Documentation Improvement Programs

Clinical Documentation Improvement (CDI) programs are not new concepts in either the medical industry or the behavioral health industry. In fact, many regulatory agencies require behavioral health organizations to have a CDI program in place. At the very least, another program could be in place called a CQI Program: a Continuous Quality Improvement Program. When preparing clinicians for the workforce, helping them to know what to expect regarding CDI is essential. Additionally, if the workplace does not happen to have a CDI program in place, then your students can be champions for helping improve documentation, and, ultimately, the standards of care. CDI programs also help mitigate risk and are often a part of an effective compliance program.

However, engendering a culture of compliance and improvement is sometimes very difficult to do within human service organizations. Some staff may be resistant to CDI programs for any variety of reasons while others will embrace the opportunity to learn and improve. Generational differences between workforce members reveal different work ethics and attitudes about what work means to the employee. Setting the tone for the program and the culture of opportunity for growth are imperative for success. The phrase "tone at the top" has been used to describe cultures where every member of the workforce is empowered to help the organization improve on its mission, values, and goals. If the executive leadership has a tone of respect, vision, and support then the workforce will be more likely to buy into the environment of trust and collaboration. It is up to leadership to set the "tone at the top," throughout the organization, and through consensus building.

CDI programs also need a tone and culture of process improvement versus a rigid, rules-based approach. Clinicians are much less defensive and open to feedback about how to improve when the tenure of the interaction is one focused on providing high-quality care to clients and on self-improvement as a professional. In addition to working towards compliance with the regulatory and payer segments, CDI programs also help improve workplace efficiency over time. Efficiency and better client quality care and metrics will become apparent to those organizations who invest in building effective compliance programs that value the organization's mission.

At a high level, CDI programs typically consist of a standardized set of chart audit forms and an iterative cycle of Health Information Management (HIM) staff randomly pulling records, reviewing and completing the paperwork, and then providing the feedback to the clinical provider. This may be an incidental occurrence or an action taken to comply with a requirement. However, this defeats the purpose of building an environment of providing high-quality healthcare service delivery. Instead of an incidental occurrence, an effective compliance program will have an internal auditing and monitoring process in place, inclusive of an internal auditing group which is continually helping clinicians improve their work documentation. Some organizations will conduct "peer audits," where your actual peers will review your records pulled at random, fill out the required paperwork, and give you the feedback. You can have internal peer reviews, or ask fellow organizations to peer review your processes on a barter / exchange basis.

The frequency and intensity of the CDI program will be driven by the following items:

- regulatory and payer requirements;
- the compliance program of the organization;
- determination of what constitutes best practices.

CDI programs are extremely effective in reviewing ICD-10-CM documentation compliance and requirements. While the ICD-10-CM items should not be the sole focus of the review, it is very easy to incorporate ICD-10 coding and documentation compliance items into the regular internal self-audits conducted by organizations, and to make this a regular occurrence.

Compliance Topics Related to the ICD and DSM

The area of policies and procedures is a large topic but for the purposes of this chapter, we will focus on only the following as they relate to the ICD and DSM topics of this book:

- clinical policies and procedures
- coding and billing policies and procedures
- administrative policies and procedures
- compliance programs.

Clinical Policies and Procedures

Throughout this text, we have discussed the need for certain policies and procedures to help guide the clinician when they are confronted with the concurrent utilization of two discrepant manuals. Generally speaking, policies and procedures are essential to demonstrate that the clinician or healthcare system has made a commitment to compliance, and to mitigate risk. Organizations will likely have a Compliance Program (CP) in place that oversees a number of processes within the organization. Small group practices are also encouraged to establish some degree of a compliance program with policies and procedures. Why? Among the rationales, a CP:

- is mandated by the Affordable Care Act of 2010 (see discussion below on compliance programs) for *all* healthcare professionals regardless of practice size *if* they accept Medicare, Medicaid, or Children's Health Insurance Plan (CHIP) funding;
- demonstrates to outside entities and all stakeholders the commitment to best practices;
- illustrates your mission to improving the quality of services delivered;
- sets the tone and both internal and external expectations of the entity;
- shows your obligation to the public, the organization/co-workers, and to the profession;
- helps provide clear, concise, and consistent information about business processes;
- mitigates risk and may actually produce cost savings if/when an audit or investigation is commenced.

There are different types of policies and procedures within an organization: administrative, clinical, fiscal, records (health information) management, staffing/workforce, HIPAA, non-retaliation, conflicts/gifts/entertainment, confidentiality, and electronic communications, to name a few. Policies and procedures are part of an effective compliance program and are put into place to address specific areas of risk. They are clear, concise, communicated, and readily available to the workforce.

Clinical policies and procedures in behavioral health organizations usually revolve around regulatory or accreditation requirements and laws such as HIPAA. As we have seen from this book, there are a number of risk areas for organizations regarding coding, documenting, billing, claims submissions and diagnosing, whether according to the DSM-series and/or the ICD series. Clinical judgment and even differing approaches to clinical practice (e.g. psychoanalytic versus CBT versus EBP) will likely vary, and may be best left "unstructured" without a policy or procedure. Once policies and procedures are formalized and implemented, however, there is an expectation that they will be shared with the workforce, followed, and updated on a regular basis. Nevertheless, policies and procedures still need to incorporate some flexibility for clinical judgment or treatment approaches.

But when it comes to the basic tenet of "How do we arrive at a diagnosis, support it, justify it, and defend it?" the different diagnostic manuals can be a source of confusion, clashing opinions, and different practices. That is even more reason for why it is important that any entity engaged in providing behavioral health services must develop a clinical policy and procedure for utilization of the two disparate, but concurrently mandated, manuals: the ICD and DSM.

Two sample templates for such a policy and procedure can be found in the Appendix. Using these as guides, you can develop a clinical policy and procedures that best fit your needs. Keep in mind that different stakeholders may require utilization of both manuals concurrently, or may just choose one. Simply stated, it is important to help clinicians navigate by providing a standard policy and procedure.

Coding, Billing Policies and Procedures

In addition to having a policy regarding the utilization of diagnostic classification manuals, every behavioral health organization needs to have a coding and billing manual or policies as well. This is essential for compliance with CMS and the OIG's fraud, waste, and abuse programs. Some organizations will have very detailed manuals for coding, documentation, and billing processes, typically called "Uniform Service Coding Standards Manuals"; on the other hand, smaller provider entities may not have these documents but instead may simply have a robust policy and procedure document(s).

Key elements for these policies, or documents, include:

- definitions of programs, provider types, and covered diagnoses;
- instructions on utilization of the different codes for billing and reimbursement: CPT, modifiers, place of service, evaluation and management, and timed codes;
- billing guidelines;
- documentation requirements.

One of the challenges for behavioral health is shoring up undefined or inconsistent business practices around coding, documentation, and billing. As pointed out in Chapter 2, there are a variety of processes that behavioral health providers use when submitting diagnoses and claims (e.g. clinician submits diagnosis directly on claim via the EHR; or clinician submits DSM diagnosis on a charge-sheet to the billing office who then converts to an ICD diagnosis;

etc.). In order to work in tandem with the medical industry to provide comprehensive, holistic care, behavioral health clinicians must be prepared to assume the responsibilities that correlate with that goal.

Unfortunately, complications abound in relation to this goal. Resources are needed to provide a higher standard of coding, documentation, and billing compliance. Formal compliance programs in behavioral health are difficult to resource, and many organizations still have not performed the risk assessment required by various mandates. Yet reimbursement rates for behavioral health services, and the traditional nature of the non-profit status itself for most human service provider entities, place behavioral health organizations at a disadvantage. Narrow operating budgets, so critically dependent on states and Medicaid programs, do not give some behavioral health providers much financial wiggle room for process improvement.

Regulatory requirements and differing, ever-changing state Medicaid rules and business processes also challenge behavioral health. Keeping abreast of the ongoing changes and implementing them throughout the business processes is time consuming and challenging. For example, consider all the custom-made, state-regulated forms in your EHR system. When there is a regulatory change, all those forms must also be updated. Workarounds or bridging gaps can put organizations at risk. This is why standardizing and formalizing many of our clinical and business processes is so important to fiscal health and true integration with all healthcare systems. Further, healthcare reform in the USA is really encouraging the behavioral health industry in the direction of becoming more standardized and medical in its processes, evidenced by trends towards value-based reimbursements, the focus on population health, and pay-for-performance models.

Administrative Policies and Procedures

Administrative Policies and Procedures, related to ICD-10-CM, involve the following categories:

- training and education
- monitoring and auditing procedures.

Both of the above items are considered "structural policies" because they guide how a program will operate. Distinct from these are "substantive policies," that define applicable regulations and how to apply them (e.g. HIPAA and the Affordable Care Act of 2010). There are a number of tangential topics in this category to take into consideration, which will not be addressed directly in this text; they are:

- establishment of an effective compliance program;
- setting up an effective, and thorough, investigations process and flow;
- correlated applicable policies including a non-retaliation policy;
- for non-profits with boards of directors: oversight of the board, board compliance and audit committees, and their duties, roles, and functions;
- whistle-blowing, *qui tam* cases, and the CMS fraud, waste, and abuse program;
- data privacy, security, and records management.

Training and Education

The training and education program is an ongoing program within the compliance program. Many organizations also have an "onboarding" process for new employees and this will need to have a section that addresses the ICD and DSM issues. Since graduate schools are only now beginning to teach the ICD series, odds are likely that there are many seasoned practicing clinicians that have never been taught the ICD series or corresponding guidelines. In fact, a recent graduate of a master's or doctoral program is more likely to understand, be knowledgeable about, and apply the ICD format than their supervisor in the workforce.

The components covered in any ICD-DSM training should at least include all the topics addressed in this book. However, to what degree each topic needs to be covered will be dependent on a number of variables, including:

1. the EHR or HIT system used by the workplace;
2. the clientele of the environment and the service delivery models;
3. whether or not you are providing services that are reported to third parties for reimbursements;
4. general acceptance of the DSM in the practice, including any requirements to use this manual in conjunction with the ICD series;
5. the review process for ensuring proper coding and documentation;
6. the culture and requirements of the workplace in acknowledging the importance of the ICD series, providing whole-person care, and assigning all applicable diagnoses (including medical and self-harm) in the medical record.

Monitoring and Auditing Processes

With respect to monitoring and auditing for coding and documentation compliance, there needs to be a standardized flow, or process, for reviewing whether or not the coding and documentation requirements are being met within an organization or practice. This ideally takes the form of a formal internal auditing process within the organization. This review process needs to be open, transparent, and discussed during the training and education stage so that everyone knows what to expect. While every organization or practice may have slightly different processes in place for conducting these reviews, the majority of healthcare entities already have such a process in place. The recommendation is to simply add, to the already-existing process, the category of coding and documentation to the regular clinical chart audits.

While there are essentially two types of audit, they could be subdivided into four different varieties: baseline-retrospective and/or concurrent-prospective audits. Baseline audits are a systemic inspection process of the records with the goal of establishing a benchmark comparison for future audits. In a sense, these audits are done for the first time and used as a template for future audits and improvements. They could be performed as retrospective audits. Retrospective audits involve reviewing entire records and itemizing the things in the record that need corrections or fixes. The challenge with retrospective audits is that if you uncover any items that require corrective action (such as overpayments), then you must remedy those actions. This will sometimes involve paybacks if overpayments are discovered, or other forms of self-reporting.

Concurrent audits are ongoing, regular reviews of the medical records and actually position the healthcare entity in a proactive position rather than a reactive state. For example, regular ongoing peer reviews or concurrent audits will identify areas needed for improvement, not corrective action. These areas for improvement or alteration are brought to the clinician's attention and can therefore be learning opportunities to improve record-keeping. This is sometimes also referred to as a "continuous quality improvement" initiative.

Finally, prospective audits are when claims are held from submission for a short period of time, about 3–7 days. During this time, the audit's objective is to make sure the clinician's documentation supports the information on the claim form, such as the CPT code, diagnosis, modifiers, and procedures (if applicable). Prospective audits ensure that clean, valid, and non-fraudulent claims are subsequently submitted to the third party.

Specifically, the monitoring and auditing process should ensure that all practitioners are using a standardized, systematized-coding, diagnostic, and documentation approach for ICD-compliance. Among the questions to be answered in this process are:

- Does the documentation support the diagnosis assigned or addressed for that healthcare encounter?
- Are the required documentation elements present in the record to back up the treating diagnosis?
- If an Unspecified or Other diagnosis is used, does it meet the CMS criteria for assigning those diagnoses?
- Are the ICD-10-CM Official Guidelines for Coding and Documentation being followed?
- Is there a consistent and standardized clinical diagnostic approach to itemizing the signs and symptoms, such as using the ICD-10 CDDG or the DSM?
- To what degree are self-harm, suicidal/homicidal ideation, medical, and all other pertinent diagnoses being coded in the record to fully describe the diagnostic picture for the case?
- Are these other diagnoses being consistently applied and are they consistent with agency policy?
- Are laterality and the other documentation elements suggested by AHIMA being applied to the medical record to substantiate medical necessity?
- In an EHR, to what degree is the copy-and-paste function being used, and is this consistent with policy?
- Is the clinician using the ICD series specifiers and corresponding digits for the diagnosis, or just notating them in the text/narrative portion of the record?

Other key areas to monitor and audit for effecting ICD-10-CM are:

Abbreviations: approved/standardized versus unapproved abbreviations	Misspellings of medications, wrong dosages documented	Misspelling or transposition of client names
Demographic errors, wrong client, wrong narrative	Persistent use of outdated modes of clinical diagnoses, such as using the five Axes of the old DSM-IV-TR	Inconsistent use of abbreviations or other frequently used items

Compliance Programs

Section 6401 of The Patient Protection and Affordable Care Act (PPACA) signed by President Obama in March of 2010 mandates that healthcare professionals establish a CP in their offices, practices, and organizations if they participate in Medicare, Medicaid, or the Children's Health Insurance Program. This means that even if you are in a state that subcontracts its Medicaid services out to a third party, if the funding comes "in part or all" from the state, which receives money from the federal government for this purpose, you must have a CP in place. CMS has numerous resources for clinicians and organizations to help them begin the process of setting up and running these programs.

Class Discussion: Who Needs a Compliance Program?

According to the PPACA of 2010, healthcare professionals are required to establish a compliance program in their offices, practices, and organizations if they participate in Medicare, Medicaid, or the CHIP.

Compliance programs, and even the application of certain HIPAA standards, are considered to be "scalable," which means the practice of due diligence and/or programs can be proportional to the size of the practice. Who decides what is considered scalable for your practice? What if your idea differs from the regulatory bodies who can sanction you? How do you determine what is industry best practice?

Does this apply to: the large community mental health center, the substance use facility, the inpatient psychiatric hospital, the sole practitioner who sees ten clients per week, or even the small group practice with ten clinicians?

What might be the critical factor if/when you are audited by an external party in determining the penalties or corrective actions? (Hint: if you genuinely put forth efforts to comply and perform some basic elements, then this effort is considered a mitigating factor in almost all cases. If, however, your efforts are on paper only and you do not have the concrete actions to demonstrate due diligence, then this is also taken into consideration.)

However, one helpful resource for establishing an effective compliance program is the book titled *Compliance 101*, published by the Health Care Compliance Association.

In the book, the authors list the OIG's "Top 10 List of Reasons to Implement a Compliance Program." Of those reasons outlined and discussed, the following have implications for the coding and documentation area in behavioral healthcare:

1. An effective CP both preserves and enhances reputation as a trustworthy provider of healthcare.
2. CPs helps providers fulfil legal duties to third parties such as the government, payers, and regulators.
3. CPs can be cost-effective and may help mitigate financial penalties levied against a healthcare entity. Certainly, not having a CP in place puts the provider at risk for things such as HIPAA violations, the False Claims Act (FCA), and the Balanced Budget Act of 1977.

Add to the mix the concerted effort on the part of the federal government to contain fraud, waste, and abuse, especially as it relates to the Medicare and Medicaid programs. For example, every week the Health Care Compliance Association publishes a brief of regulatory actions taken (and settled with the parties) against healthcare providers. In 2016, there were on average five federal actions finalized and taken during any given week. Some of these settlements involved prison time, large payback fines and penalties, or other significant consequences meant to send a message to others and deter further violations. Cases ranged from solo practitioners to small group practices and entire healthcare systems.

In other words: no one is immune when it comes to the OIG's effort to combat fraud, waste, and abuse. The OIG publishes "OIG Most Wanted (Healthcare) Fugitives" on their website. Even third-party payers have regulatory requirements they must meet for the CMS/OIG programs to fight fraud. Third-party health plans have their own program integrity or fraud, waste, and abuse departments in order to comply with the laws. The request for records may originate with the third-party payer, but if any of the funds involved were "in part or all" sourced at the Federal CMS level, then those audit requests can go all the way to the OIG, if determined to be serious enough.

Given this brief discussion on compliance, it becomes clear that a compliance program is not only a mandate for most healthcare providers, it becomes smart business practice. The robustness of the program will be dependent on any number of factors such as agency/practice size, resources, and, most importantly, commitment to ensuring quality care that delivers value while mitigating risk.

Class Discussion

The New Mexico Fraud, Waste, and Abuse Saga

In March 2011, CMS issued bulletin CPI-B 11-04 reiterating its authority to enforce the PPACA by suspending Medicaid funding to healthcare entities when there are "credible allegations of fraud."

In June of 2013, the New Mexico Human Services Department retained the auditing group Public Consulting Group (PCG) to conduct audits of 15 behavioral healthcare providers across the state of New Mexico. Between those 15 agencies, approximately 30,000 consumers with serious mental illness were receiving services from those agencies. The New Mexico Human Service Department notified the provider agencies that there were "credible allegations of fraud for which an investigation is pending" and this enabled them to suspend all Medicaid payments to these provider organizations.

Concurrently, officials in New Mexico began to contract with provider organizations in neighboring Arizona to come in and take over operations of the agencies affected.

In July–August of 2013, eight agencies went to court to get their funding restored but they were not successful. The PCG audit results were turned over to New Mexico's State Auditor. The New Mexico Legislature also got involved and denied funding to bring in the Arizona providers. Clearly, the clientele at these New Mexico organizations were deeply affected. Clients' care was being compromised, the New Mexico agencies and some at the state level began to question the secrecy surrounding the audits and the "results."

By September 2013, the case had reached a new height with the legal battles, lawyers from all parts of the country were getting involved, and there were calls for the release of the full audit. There was a lot of controversy over the issue because the New Mexico providers had never been told what they did wrong, other than that there were findings of "fraud."

In the Fall of 2013, a heavily redacted partial audit was released but this did not assuage feelings or answer the questions. Instead, the partial audit release revealed that the 15 provider organizations were "overpaid by 36 million dollars over three years." The newspaper *Las Cruces Sun News* unsuccessfully filed a lawsuit seeking disclosure of the full audit based on the Inspection of Public Records Act. The challenges and legal proceedings continued.

In January 2015, a new State Attorney General for New Mexico took over the reins, and released the audit in full. At this point in time, it was revealed that *the New Mexico Department of Human Services had removed a sentence on page 22 of the 400-page report written by PCG that "it had found no 'credible allegations of fraud'."* Further, the allegations of fraud amounted not to 36 million dollars but to $42,500 across all 15 provider organizations.

It took until February of 2016 for the New Mexico Attorney General to *exonerate* ten of the 15 healthcare provider organizations. Two of the organizations had settled in order to continue their operations. Some organizations that had closed never reopened, leaving their clientele in a difficult situation.

Do you know what constitutes a credible allegation of fraud? Look up the CMS Bulletin CPI-B 11-04 to find out!

- Do you think the regulators look only at the financial impact of state and federal funding, such as overpayments or false claims? What else might they look at?
- If you do not chart your session note on the session that you just performed, how might regulators look at this within the framework of fraud, waste, and abuse?
- How do regulators determine a healthcare encounter actually occurred if there are no session notes?
- If you were a regulator, what would you look for?

One of the most overlooked areas of any effective CP is that of risk assessment. In fact, the 2016 OIG Work Plan has indicated that it is going to take a close look at selected entities' compliance with the mandated risk assessments outlined in HIPAA and in other regulations. Healthcare data breaches affecting more than 500 individuals are to be reported to the Office of Civil Rights (OCR). When the breaches are reported, and the subsequent investigations take place, many provider organizations are found not only to have suffered a breach, but also to have not even conducted the mandated baseline risk assessment. Unfortunately, that additional finding just doubled the organization's problems. While coding and documentation are areas that are not typically covered in most risk assessments, they should be a part of any organization's compliance program, ongoing internal monitoring and auditing, and ensuing risk management program.

Summary

Coding and documentation are critical elements of billing, reimbursements, healthcare encounters, client safety, and the provision of high-quality healthcare service delivery. Keep in mind that coding and documentation compliance in behavioral healthcare is not optional, but is a requirement and mandated by CMS, HIPAA, regulatory and accrediting bodies, and state laws. The task for behavioral health clinicians is to find a way to integrate our long history and tradition of providing healthcare services that differ from the medical sciences, yet play a pivotal role in improving population health. To be mindful that medical, social, and psychological needs frequently go hand-in-hand, we must code and document accurately, thoroughly, and in a way that promotes a holistic picture in our endeavors to achieve the triple aim: improving the patient experience of healthcare, improving health populations, and reducing the per capita cost of healthcare.

To recap the essential points:

1. Compliance with the ICD-10-CM is not optional in the USA if you are a HIPAA-covered entity. This means more than just assigning the right diagnostic code. It means knowing the coding and documentation guidelines and putting processes in place that ensure all coding and documentation meet the regulatory requirements.
2. CMS is really the key in leadership for knowing what and how to document in the medical records. CMS produces a number of helpful "Provider Bulletins" to keep the industry abreast of new or updated regulations and also of best practices.
3. The burden is on the clinician or provider organization to train and educate their staff on the utilization of ICD-10-CM in a way that maintains standardization, consistency, and fidelity to the healthcare industry at large.
4. The establishment of a compliance program has been mandated by the Affordable Care Act of 2010 if any revenues received come in part, or all, from the state Medicaid agency. There are essential elements of processes

that constitute an effective compliance program, including performing risk assessments, and ongoing monitoring and auditing of business processes.

Bibliography

American Health Information Management Association. (2005, April). *Documentation and Reimbursement for Behavioral Healthcare Services.* Chicago, IL: American Health Information Management Association.

American Medical Association. (2009). *Current Procedural Terminology: CPT.* Chicago, IL: American Medical Association.

Centers for Medicare & Medicaid Services. (2009, June 5). Revised appendix A, "Interpretive guidelines for hospitals." CMS Manual System, Pub. 100-07 State Operations Provider Certification (47). Retrieved April 16, 2016 from www.cms.gov/Regulations-and-Guidance/Guidance/Transmittals/downloads/R47SOMA.pdf.

Centers for Medicare & Medicaid Services. (2011, March 25). CPI – CMCS informational bulletin: Affordable Care Act program integrity provisions – Guidance to states – Section 6402(h)(2) – Suspension of Medicaid payments based upon pending investigations of credible allegations of fraud, CPI-B 11-04. Retrieved April 15, 2016 from http://oig.hhs.gov/fraud/medicaid-fraud-control-units-mfcu/files/payment-suspensions-info-bulletin-3-25-2011.pdf.

Centers for Medicare & Medicaid Services. (2012). Conditions of Participation: Medical Record Services, 42 CFR 482.24.

Centers for Medicare & Medicaid Services. (2015, December). Medicaid documentation for behavioral health practitioners. Retrieved April 15, 2016 from www.cms.gov/Medicare-Medicaid-Coordination/Fraud-Prevention/Medicaid-Integrity-Education/Downloads/docmatters-behavioralhealth-factsheet.pdf.

Comfort, A., & Endicott, M. (2014, December 10). *CMS and AHIMA Webinar: ICD-10 and Clinical Documentation* [PowerPoint Slides]. Retrieved May 16, 2015 from file:///C:/Users/RichardAndLaura/Downloads/CMS%20and%20AHIMA%20ICD-10%20Clinical%20Documentation%20Webinar%202014-12-10%20(1).pdf.

Institute for Healthcare Improvement. (2016). *The IHI Triple Aim.* Retrieved April 16, 2016 from www.ihi.org/engage/initiatives/tripleaim/pages/default.aspx.

Substance Abuse and Mental Health Services Administration Center for Substance Abuse Treatment. (2006). *Addiction Counseling Competencies: The Knowledge, Skills, and Attitudes of Professional Practice.* Technical Assistance Publication (TAP) Series 21. Retrieved April 16, 2016 from http://store.samhsa.gov/shin/content//SMA12-4171/SMA12-4171.pdf.

Substance Abuse and Mental Health Services Administration – Health Resources and Services Administration Center for Integrated Health Solutions. (2014, January). *Core Competencies for Integrated Behavioral Health and Primary Care.* Retrieved February 19, 2016 from www.integration.samhsa.gov/workforce/Integration_Competencies_Final.pdf.

Taitsman, J., Culbertson, J.D., & Bloink, J. (2014). *Affordable Care Act Provider Compliance Programs: Getting Started Webinar* [PowerPoint Slides]. Retrieved April 15, 2016 from www.cms.gov/Outreach-and-Education/Medicare-Learning-Network-MLN/MLNEdWebGuide/Downloads/MLN-Compliance-Webinar.pdf.

Troklus, D., & Warner, G. (2011). *Compliance 101*, 3rd edn. Minneapolis, MN: Health Care Compliance Association.

Disclaimer

The items in the Appendices which follow are for guidance purposes only. Please note these are samples from a variety of sources and serve as suggestions only. You are responsible for the content of any Appendix item you choose to use or edit, and for any diagnosis or diagnosis-related item you assign or use.

Final formatting of the Appendices attempted to replicate the handouts as given to audiences. Appendix A, a one-page Excel spreadsheet, may not be reflected as such in the ebook version due to electronic formatting constraints. Appendix B is also an Excel spreadsheet that is affected by the constraints of electronic formatting.

Substance Use Table A

This table was created by Angela Hickman. Please be advised that it is the clinician's responsibility to

		Uncomp	In remission	Delirium	Perceptual disturbance	Unspec
Alcohol						
Abuse		F10.10				
w/intoxication		F10.120		F10.121		F10.129
w/induced psychotic disorder						F10.159
w/other induced disorders						F10.19
Dependence		F10.20	F10.21			
w/intoxication		F10.220		F10.221		F10.229
w/withdrawal		F10.230		F10.231	F10.232	F10.239
w/induced psychotic disorder						F10.259
w/persisting amnestic disorder	F10.26					
w/persisting dementia	F10.27					
w/other induced disorders						F10.29
Use						
w/intoxication		F10.920		F10.921		F10.929
w/induced psychotic disorder						F10.959
w/persisting amnestic disorder	F10.96					
w/persisting dementia	F10.97					
w/other induced disorders						F10.99
Opioid						
Abuse		F11.10				
w/intoxication		F11.120		F11.121	F11.122	F11.129
w/induced psychotic disorder						F11.159
w/other induced disorders						F11.19
Dependence		F11.20	F11.21			
w/intoxication		F11.220		F11.221	F11.222	F11.229
w/withdrawal	F11.23					
w/induced psychotic disorder	F11.25					F11.259
w/other induced disorders						F11.29
Use		F11.90				
w/intoxication		F11.920		F11.921	F11.922	F11.929
w/induced psychotic disorder						F11.959
w/other induced disorders						F11.99
w/withdrawl	F11.93					

© 2017, *Coding and Documentation Compliance for the ICD and DSM*, Wright, Tobias, Hickman, Routledge.

assign the appropriate diagnosis and to verify the code number used is congruent with the FY Tabular Index.

W/induced mood disorder	**W/ delusions**	**W/ hallucinations**	**W/induced anxiety disorder**	**W/induced sexual dysfunction**	**W/induced sleep disorder**	**W/other induced disorder**
F10.14						
	F10.150	F10.151				
			F10.180	F10.181	F10.182	F10.188
F10.24						
	F10.250	F10.251				
			F10.280	F10.281	F10.282	F10.288
F10.94						
	F10.950	F10.951				
			F10.980	F10.981	F10.982	F10.988
F11.14						
	F11.150	F11.151				
				F11.181	F11.182	F11.188
F11.24						
	F11.250	F11.251				
				F11.281	F11.282	F11.288
F11.94						
	F11.950	F11.951				
				F11.981	F11.982	F11.988

© 2017, *Coding and Documentation Compliance for the ICD and DSM*, Wright, Tobias, Hickman, Routledge.

This table was created by Angela Hickman. Please be advised that it is the clinician's responsibility to

		Uncomp	In remission	Delirium	Perceptual disturbance	Unspec
Cannabis						
Abuse		F12.10				
w/intoxication		F12.120		F12.121	F12.122	F12.129
w/induced psychotic disorder						F12.159
w/other induced disorders						F12.19
Dependence		F12.20	F12.21			
w/intoxication		F12.220		F12.221	F12.222	F12.229
w/induced psychotic disorder						F12.259
w/other induced disorders						F12.29
Use		F12.90				
w/intoxication		F12.920		F12.921	F12.922	F12.929
w/induced psychotic disorder						F12.929
w/other induced disorders						F12.99
Sedative, hypnotic, or anxiolytic						
Abuse		F13.10				
w/intoxication		F13.120		F13.121		F13.129
w/induced psychotic disorder						F13.59
w/other induced disorders						F13.19
Dependence		F13.20	F13.21			
w/intoxication		F13.220		F13.221		F13.229
w/withdrawal		F13.230		F13.231	F13.232	F13.239
w/induced psychotic disorder						F13.259
w/persisting amnestic disorder	F13.26					
w/persisting dementia	F13.27					
w/other induced disorders						F13.29
Use		F13.90				
w/intoxication		F13.920		F13.921		F13.929
w/withdrawal		F13.930		F13.931	F13.932	F13.939
w/induced psychotic disorder						F13.959
w/persisting amnestic disorder	F13.96					
w/persisting dementia	F13.97					
w/other induced disorders						F13.99

© 2017, *Coding and Documentation Compliance for the ICD and DSM*, Wright, Tobias, Hickman, Routledge.

assign the appropriate diagnosis and to verify the code number used is congruent with the FY Tabular Index.

W/induced mood disorder	W/ delusions	W/ hallucinations	W/induced anxiety disorder	W/induced sexual dysfunction	W/induced sleep disorder	W/other induced disorder
	F12.150	F12.151				
			F12.180			F12.188
	F12.250	F12.251				
			F12.280			F12.288
	F12.950	F12.951				
			F12.980			F12.988
F13.14						
	F13.150	F13.151				
			F13.180	F13.181	F13.182	F13.188
F13.24						
	F13.250	F13.251				
			F13.280	F13.281	F13.282	F13.288
F13.94						
	F13.950	F13.951				
			F13.980	F13.981	F13.982	F13.988

© 2017, *Coding and Documentation Compliance for the ICD and DSM*, Wright, Tobias, Hickman, Routledge.

This table was created by Angela Hickman. Please be advised that it is the clinician's responsibility to

		Uncomp	In remission	Delirium	Perceptual disturbance	Unspec
Cocaine						
Abuse		F14.10				
w/intoxication		F14.120		F14.121	F14.122	F14.129
w/induced psychotic disorder						F14.159
w/other induced disorders						F14.19
Dependence		F14.20	F14.21			
w/intoxication		F14.220		F14.221	F14.222	F14.229
w/withdrawal	F14.23					
w/induced psychotic disorder						F14.259
w/other induced disorders						F14.29
Use		F14.90				
w/intoxication		F14.920		F14.921	F14.922	F14.929
w/withdrawal						
w/induced psychotic disorder						F14.959
w/other induced disorders						F14.99
Other stimulant						
Abuse		F15.10				
w/intoxication		F15.120		F15.121	F15.122	F15.129
w/induced psychotic disorder						F15.159
w/other induced disorders						F15.19
Dependence		F15.20	F15.21			
w/intoxication		F15.220		F15.221	F15.222	F15.229
w/withdrawal	F15.23					
w/induced psychotic disorder						F15.259
w/other induced disorders						F15.29
Use		F15.90				
w/intoxication		F15.920		F15.921	F15.922	F15.929
w/withdrawal	F15.93					
w/induced psychotic disorder						
w/other induced disorders						F15.99
Hallucinogenics						
Abuse		F16.10				
w/intoxication		F16.120		F16.121	F16.122	F16.129
w/induced psychotic disorder						F16.159
w/other induced disorders						F16.19
w/perception disorder (flashbacks)	F16.183					

© 2017, *Coding and Documentation Compliance for the ICD and DSM*, Wright, Tobias, Hickman, Routledge.

assign the appropriate diagnosis and to verify the code number used is congruent with the FY Tabular Index.

W/induced mood disorder	W/ delusions	W/ hallucinations	W/induced anxiety disorder	W/induced sexual dysfunction	W/induced sleep disorder	W/other induced disorder
F14.14						
	F14.150	F14.151				
			F14.180	F14.181	F14.182	F14.188
F14.24						
	F14.250	F14.251				
			F14.280	F14.281	F14.282	F14.288
F14.94						
	F14.950	F14.951				
			F14.980	F14.981	F14.982	F14.988
F15.14						
	F15.150	F15.151				
			F15.180	F15.181	F15.182	F15.188
F15.24						
	F15.250	F15.251				
			F15.280	F15.281	F15.282	F15.288
F15.94						
F15.959	F15.950	F15.951				
			F15.980	F15.981	F15.982	F15.988
F16.14						
	F16.150	F16.151				
			F16.180			F16.188

© 2017, *Coding and Documentation Compliance for the ICD and DSM*, Wright, Tobias, Hickman, Routledge.

This table was created by Angela Hickman. Please be advised that it is the clinician's responsibility to

		Uncomp	In remission	Delirium	Perceptual disturbance	Unspec
Dependence		F16.20	F16.21			
w/intoxication		F16.220		F16.221		F16.229
w/induced psychotic disorder						F16.259
w/other induced disorders						F16.29
w/perception disorder (flashbacks)	F16.283					
Use		F16.90				
w/intoxication		F16.920		F16.921		F16.929
w/induced psychotic disorder						F16.959
w/other induced disorders						F16.99
w/perception disorder (flashbacks)	F16.983					
Other psychoactive						
Abuse		F19.10				
w/intoxication		F19.120		F19.121	F19.122	F19.129
w/induced psychotic disorder						F19.159
w/persisting amnestic disorder	F19.16					
w/persisting dementia	F19.17					
w/other induced disorders						F19.19
Dependence		F19.20	F19.21			
w/intoxication		F19..220		F19.221	F19.222	F19.229
w/withdrawal		F19.230		F19.231	F19.232	F19.239
w/induced psychotic disorder						F19.259
w/persisting amnestic disorder	F19.26					
w/persisting dementia	F19.27					
w/other induced disorders						F19.29
Use		F19.90				
w/intoxication		F19.920		F19.921	F19.922	F19.929
w/withdrawal		F19.930		F19.931	F19.932	F19.939
w/induced psychotic disorder						F19.959
w/persisting amnestic disorder	F19.96					
w/persisting dementia	F19.97					
w/other induced disorders						F19.99

© 2017, *Coding and Documentation Compliance for the ICD and DSM*, Wright, Tobias, Hickman, Routledge.

assign the appropriate diagnosis and to verify the code number used is congruent with the FY Tabular Index.

W/induced mood disorder	W/ delusions	W/ hallucinations	W/induced anxiety disorder	W/induced sexual dysfunction	W/induced sleep disorder	W/other induced disorder
F16.24						
	F16.250	F16.251				
			F16.280			F16.288
F16.94						
	F16.950	F16.951				
			F16.980			F16.988
F19.14						
	F19.150	F19.151				
			F19.180	F19.181	F19.182	F19.188
F19.24						
	F19.250	F19.251				
			F19.280	F19.281	F19.282	F19.288
F19.94						
	F19.950	F19.951				
			F19.980	F19.981	F19.982	F19.988

© 2017, *Coding and Documentation Compliance for the ICD and DSM*, Wright, Tobias, Hickman, Routledge.

B

Sample ICD-10 Documentation Requirements Table

This document was created and compiled by Angela Hickman. Any diagnosis given to a client acurracy of all codes utilized.

FY 2017 ICD-10-CM DOCUMENTATION REQUIREMENTS

ICD-9-CM CODE	ICD-9-CM CODE DESCRIPTION	ICD-10 CODE CATEGORY	ICD-10-CM CODE CATEGORY DESCRIPTION	ICD-10-CM SPECIFIED CODE CONDITION/ DISEASE
278.00	Obesity, unspecified	E66.9	Obesity, unspecified	Obesity
300.00	Anxiety state, unspecified	F41.1	Generalized anxiety disorder	Generalized anxiety disorder
300.4	Dysthymic disorder	F34.1	Dysthymic disorder	Dysthymic disorder
250.00	Diabetes Mellitus	E08-E13.9	Diabetes Mellitus	Diabetes Mellitus
311	Depressive disorder, not elsewhere classified	F32.9	Depressive disorder NOS	Depressive disorder
296.22	Major depressive disorder, single episode, moderate	F32.1		
296.23	Major depressive disorder, single episode, severe, without mention of psychotic behavior	F32.2		
314.00	Attention-deficit disorder of childhood without mention of hyperactivity	F90.0	ADHD, predominantly inattentive type	Attention-deficit disorders

© 2017, *Coding and Documentation Compliance for the ICD and DSM*, Wright, Tobias, Hickman, Routledge.

is the responsibility of the clinician assigning the diagnosis. You are responsible for verifying the

ICD-10-CM SPECIFIED CODE(S) CATEGORY	ICD-10-CM CODE CATEGORY DESCRIPTION	REQUIRED DOCUMENTATION
E66.01	Morbid (severe) obesity due to excess calories	1. Type: morbid (severe) obesity due to excess calories, other due to excess calories, drug-induced, morbid (severe) with alveolar hypoventilation, overweight, other, unspecified 2. Indicate: obesity complicating pregnancy, childbirth, puerperium, BMI, if known, drug, if applicable
E66.09	Other obesity due to excess calories	
E66.1	Drug-induced obesity	
E66.2	Morbid (severe) obesity with alveolar hypoventilation	
E66.3	Overweight	
E66.8	Other obesity	
E66.9	Obesity, unspecified	
F41.1	Generalized anxiety disorder	1. Type (anxiety neurosis, anxiety reaction, anxiety state, overanxious disorder)
F34.1	Dysthymic disorder	1. Type (depressive neurosis, depressive personality disorder, dysthymia, neurotic depression, persistent anxiety depression)
E08–E13.9	Diabetes Mellitus	1. Type: type 1, type 2, drug induced, other specified, etc. 2. Complications 3. Manifestations 4. Insulin use 5. Body system affected 6. Secondary
F32.0	Major depressive disorder, single episode, mild	1. Type (major depressive disorder) 2. Indicate: single episode, recurrent, mild, moderate, severe without psychotic features, severe with psychotic features, severe with psychotic symptoms 3. Remission, partial, full, unspecified
F32.1	Major depressive disorder, single episode, moderate	
F32.2	Major depressive disorder, single episode, severe without psychotic features	
F32.3	Major depressive disorder, single episode, severe with psychotic features	
F90.0	Attention-deficit hyperactivity disorder, predominantly inattentive type	Type: predominantly inattentive, predominatly hyperactive, combined, other, unspecified

© 2017, *Coding and Documentation Compliance for the ICD and DSM*, Wright, Tobias, Hickman, Routledge.

This document was created and compiled by Angela Hickman. Any diagnosis given to a client acurracy of all codes utilized.

FY 2017 ICD-10-CM DOCUMENTATION REQUIREMENTS

ICD-9-CM CODE	ICD-9-CM CODE DESCRIPTION	ICD-10 CODE CATEGORY	ICD-10-CM CODE CATEGORY DESCRIPTION	ICD-10-CM SPECIFIED CODE CONDITION/ DISEASE
314.01	Attention deficit disorder of childhood with hyperactivity	F90.1	Attention-deficit hyperactivity disorder, predominantly hyperactive type	
314.1	Hyperkinesis of childhood with developmental delay	F90.8		
303.90	Other and unspecified alcohol dependence, unspecified	F10.20	Alcohol dependence, uncomplicated	Alcohol dependence
290.42	Vascular dementia, with delusions	F01.51	Vascular dementia with behavioral disturbance	Vascular dementia
309.81	Post-traumatic stress disorder	F43.10	Post-traumatic stress disorder, unspecified	Post-traumatic stress disorder (PTSD)

© 2017, *Coding and Documentation Compliance for the ICD and DSM*, Wright, Tobias, Hickman, Routledge.

is the responsibility of the clinician assigning the diagnosis. You are responsible for verifying the

ICD-10-CM SPECIFIED CODE(S) CATEGORY	ICD-10-CM CODE CATEGORY DESCRIPTION	REQUIRED DOCUMENTATION
F90.1	Attention-deficit hyperactivity disorder, predominantly hyperactive type	
F90.2	Attention-deficit hyperactivity disorder, combined type	
F90.8	Attention-deficit hyperactivity disorder, other type	
F90.9	Attention-deficit hyperactivity disorder, unspecified type	
F10.20	Alcohol dependence, uncomplicated	1. With: intoxication, withdrawal mood disorder, psychotic disorder, persisting amnestic disorder, persisting dementia, other alcohol-induced disorders, unspecified alcohol-induced disorder
F10.21	Alcohol dependence, in remission	
F10.220-F10.229	Alcohol dependence with intoxication	2. Identify: uncomplicated, in remission, with delirium, with perceptual disturbance, with delusions, with hallucinations, with anxiety disorder, with sexual dysfunction, with sleep disorder, with unspecified disorder
F10.230-F10.239	Alcohol dependence with withdrawal	
F10.24	Alcohol dependence with alcohol-induced mood disorder	
F10.250-F10.259	Alcohol dependence with alcohol-induced psychotic disorder	
F10.26	Alcohol dependence with alochol-induced persisting amnestic disorder	
F10.27	Alcohol dependence with alcohol-induced persisting dementia	
F10.280-F10.288	Alcohol dependence with other alcohol-induced disorders	
F10.29	Alcohol dependence with unspecified alcohol-induced disorder	
F01.50	Vascular dementia without behavioral disturbance	1. Behavioral disturbance: with/without 2. Identify underlying physiological condition or sequelae of cerebrovascular disease, wandering in vascular dementia
F01.51	Vascular dementia with behavioral disturbance	
F43.10	Post-traumatic stress disorder, unspecified	1. Type: acute, chronic, unspecified
F43.11	PTSD, acute	
F43.12	PTSD, chronic	

© 2017, *Coding and Documentation Compliance for the ICD and DSM*, Wright, Tobias, Hickman, Routledge.

This document was created and compiled by Angela Hickman. Any diagnosis given to a client acurracy of all codes utilized.

FY 2017 ICD-10-CM DOCUMENTATION REQUIREMENTS

ICD-9-CM CODE	ICD-9-CM CODE DESCRIPTION	ICD-10 CODE CATEGORY	ICD-10-CM CODE CATEGORY DESCRIPTION	ICD-10-CM SPECIFIED CODE CONDITION/ DISEASE
493.00	Extrinsic asthma, unspecified	J45.909	Unspecified asthma, uncomplicated	Asthma
493.92 493.02 493.91 493.90	Asthma, unspecified, with (acute) exacerbation	J45.901, J45.902, J45.909	Unspecified asthma with (acute) exacerbation	
307.40	Nonorganic sleep disorder, unspecified	F51.9	Sleep disorder not due to a substance or known physiological condition, unspecified	Sleep disorders not due to a substance or known physiological condition

© 2017, *Coding and Documentation Compliance for the ICD and DSM*, Wright, Tobias, Hickman, Routledge.

is the responsibility of the clinician assigning the diagnosis. You are responsible for verifying the

ICD-10-CM SPECIFIED CODE(S) CATEGORY	ICD-10-CM CODE CATEGORY DESCRIPTION	REQUIRED DOCUMENTATION
J45.2-	Mild intermittent asthma	1. Type: mild intermittent, mild persistent, moderate persistent, severe persistent, exercise induced bronchospasm, cough variant, other and unspecified 2. Identify: uncomplicated, with exacerbation, with status asthmaticus 3. History of tobacco use, exposure to tobacco smoke, tobacco dependence 4. Severity
J45.3-	Mild persistent asthma	
J45.4-	Moderate persistent asthma	
J45.5-	Severe persistent asthma	
J45.9-	Other and unspecified asthma	
F51.01	Primary insomnia	1. Type: insomnia – primary, adjustment, paradoxical, psychophysiologic, due to other mental disorders, other insomnia not due to a substance or known physiological condition; Hypersomnia – primary, insufficient sleep syndrome, due to other mental disorder, other hypersomnia not due to a substance or known physiological condition, sleepwalking, sleep terrors, nightmare disorder, other sleep disorders not due to a substance or known physiological condition, sleep disorder not due to a substance or known physiological condition, unspecified 2. Identify associated mental disorder, if applicable
F51.02	Adjustment insomnia	
F51.03	Paradoxical insomnia	
F51.04	Psychophysiologic insomnia	
F51.05	Insomnia due to other mental disorder	
F51.09	Other insomnia not due to a substance or known physiological condition	
F51.11	Primary hypersomnia	
F51.12	Insufficient sleep syndrome	
F51.13	Hypersomnia due to other mental disorder	
F51.19	Other hypersomnia not due to a substance or known physiological condition	
F51.3	Sleepwalking	
F51.4	Sleep terrors	
F51.5	Nightmare disorder	
F51.8	Other sleep disorders not due to a substance	
F51.9	Sleep disorder not due to a substance or known physiological condition, unspecified	

© 2017, *Coding and Documentation Compliance for the ICD and DSM*, Wright, Tobias, Hickman, Routledge.

C

Clinical Policy Sample 1, Coding and Documentation

Policy and Scope

[NAME OF YOUR ORGANIZATION] will comply with the requirements set forth in the [NAME OF YOUR STATE] and Federal False Claims Act in an effort to prevent fraud against federal, state and local governmental entities.

Purpose

To ensure that [NAME OF YOUR ORGANIZATION] is using a standardized, systemic coding, diagnostic, and documentation approach.

Key Procedures and Provisions

1. Clinicians will be sufficiently trained in coding techniques and current coding requirements to ensure that the diagnostic codes selected accurately depict the service performed.
2. Codes for payment must correlate with the documentation in the client's medical record and comply with the particular rules associated with billing these codes.
3. We will follow the "ICD-10-CM Official Guidelines for Coding and Reporting."

4. Each client record will contain sufficient documentation to support the treating diagnosis.
5. Each client record will minimally contain the following clinical information: diagnosis documentation, pertinent history, treatment plan, progress made, response to treatment, recommendations and discharge status.
6. [You may want to put a statement in here about which diagnostic manual you will be using, for the clinical criteria (DSM versus ICD Clinical Descriptions and Diagnostic Guidelines).]
7. [You may want to put something here about where you will obtain your code numbers from, how they have been verified, approved, etc.]
8. [You may decide to add here certain compliance guidelines, or an itemization of completing certain tasks. These should be based on any regulatory standards that govern your organization, such as Joint Commission standards, e.g. "Diagnosis shall be assigned within x-hour/days."]
9. Only authorized personnel (Certified Professional Coders and Clinicians) may assign diagnosis codes based on provider documentation. Questions about a code assignment are addressed to the clinician responsible for the client.

Responsibility

The Medical Director or Clinical Director will oversee implementation of this policy to ensure that coding, documentation, and diagnosing are assigned according to the CMS and HIPAA-mandated ICD guidelines.

Clinical Policy Sample 2, Coding and Documentation

D

Policy and Scope

[YOUR NAME] is a licensed facility, governed by the [NAME OF STATE] Code, Chapters [xxx], [xxx] (Title [xxx], Health and Safety) and [NAME OF STATE] Code, Chapter [xxx]. Concurrent utilization of the ICD and DSM-5 classification systems may be mandated by CMS, HIPAA, and by [put reference here if your state mandates use of the DSM or third-party payers]. This has the potential to be confounding to clinicians who use the systems. This policy represents our approach to reconciling the two systems.

We acknowledge that the ICD is the only CMS-approved code set to be utilized for healthcare purposes that is HIPAA-compliant. We concurrently acknowledge that the DSM has been the standard classification system of mental disorders used by behavioral health professionals in the USA.

The ICD classification system has definitive dates of implementation determined by the US government. The DSM, however, is not regulated by the US government and therefore different versions of the DSM can be used at different times, for different purposes.

Purpose

The purpose of this policy is to ensure [YOUR NAME] is using the most current, up-to-date, and clinically sound best practices based on federal and state laws, coupled with the regulatory requirements of being a licensed facility in the state of [NAME OF STATE]. State licensure requirements of our clinical staff regulate the scope of practice and manner in which consumer health information is managed.

Key Procedures and Provisions

ICD/DSM Utilization

1. ICD diagnostic codes must be assigned to an individual for purposes of HIPAA, claims, and reimbursement purposes.
2. DSM diagnostic codes may be requested by some third-party payers for purposes of clinical review, documentation, or for the authorization for services. ICD codes may also be requested for this same purpose.

ICD/DSM Code Assignment

1. Only authorized personnel (Clinicians or Certified Professional Coders) may assign, and are responsible for, diagnosis codes. If there is a question about a code, the Clinician responsible for the consumer shall make the final determination to the correct code.
2. [Make a note here about your use of "other/unspecified" codes and your intent.]

ICD/DSM Language and Coding Number Discrepancies

1. There are instances of mental disorders labeled differently in the ICD than in the DSM. There are instances in which the codes and their corresponding numbers from one code set are not matched, or found, in the other set.
2. We will explain to clients, wherever possible and deemed appropriate, that the label for their condition may be titled differently by a third party.
3. If our staff become aware of a coding number and diagnosis discrepancy between the code sets, then it will be the responsibility of the clinician to clarify which code number, classification system, and diagnosis is to be used for the needed purpose.

ICD/DSM Coding and Recording Protocols

1. Both the ICD and DSM have official documentation and recording protocols mandated for use. As required, we will utilize the ICD-10-CM system "ICD-10-CM Official Guidelines for Coding and Recording." This decision is based in part on the DSM's own endorsement for utilizing the Official Guidelines for Coding and Recording.
2. If a diagnosis has two different code numbers between the manuals, the clinician will document the ICD code first, with a notation of the appropriate DSM code.
3. "Code First" refers to the DSM and ICM coding conventions requiring that any underlying medical or other etiological cause to the condition be sequenced first. Licensing and scope of practice laws limit the practice of medicine as do practice laws of other healthcare disciplines. Therefore, our staff will:

    - make a written notation in the record regarding the medical condition;
    - assign the corresponding ICD or DSM medical code as a secondary, tertiary or subsequent diagnosis;
    - assign the least specific medical diagnosis code available to account for the general condition [OR: assign 3-, 4-, 5-digit codes to medical diagnoses] [OR: use only the "Approved Medical Diagnoses" endorsed by our organization];
    - possibly assign more specific medical diagnosis codes (if this is allowed by the practitioner's scope of practice and state law).

4. "Other" refers to the ICD Coding and Documentation Guidelines that state the most specific diagnosis should be used. Using a diagnosis of "other" is reserved for those cases in which another, more specific, code does not exist, and will be supported by clinical documentation. "Unspecified" codes will be used when they meet the criteria in the coding and documentation guidelines.
5. Treatment plans: While the ICD-10 Official Coding and Documentation Guidelines indicate that a treatment plan must accompany every diagnosis given to a client, we have decided that we will have a (single) comprehensive treatment plan that is reflective of the main reason for treatment at our organization in lieu of multiple treatment plans [or some similar wording here].

Responsibility

The Clinical Director and/or Designee shall oversee implementing this policy and determine what training, remediation, or other actions must be taken to ensure compliance throughout the organization.

Cheat Sheet: Schizoaffective

E

"Cheat sheets" are designed and individualized by end users in a manner that best suits their needs. The cheat sheets in Appendixes E, F and G were designed by a group of hospital clinicians to give them useful prompts or hints as to what terms they could use in the record to support their diagnosis.

SCHIZOAFFECTIVE F25	F25.0 SCHIZOAFFECTIVE DISORDER, MANIC TYPE F25.1 SCHIZOAFFECTIVE DISORDER, DEPRESSIVE TYPE F25.2 SCHIZOAFFECIVE DISORDER, MIXED TYPE F25.9 SCHIZOAFFECTIVE DISORDER, UNSPECIFIED
Diagnostic Criteria and Guidelines • Mood swings • Labile • Mood Disturbance • Elevated Moods • Hallucinations • Anger • Posturing • Isolation • Poor Communication • Poor Relationships • Agitated • Hopeless • Helpless • Hostile • Sucidal/Homicidal Ideation	BLUE BOOK CRITERIA ONLY F25.0 – Schizoaffective Disorder, Manic Type- There must be a prominent elevation of mood, or a less obvious elevation of mood combined with increased irritability or excitement. Within the same episode, at least one and preferably two typically schizophrenic symptoms (as specified for schizophrenia (F20), diagnostic guidelines (a)–(d)) should be clearly present. This category should be used both for a single schizoaffective episode of the manic type and for a recurrent disorder in which the majority of episodes are schizoaffective, manic type.

- Dramatic
- Psychotic
- Grimaces
- Primitive
- Strange Body Gestures
- Disorganized Speech
- Bizarre
- Mutism
- Hyperverbal
- Exaggerated

F25.1 – Schizoaffective Disorder, Depressive Type

There must be prominent depression, accompanied by at least two characteristic depressive symptoms or associated behavioral abnormalities as listed for depressive episode; within the same episode, at least one and preferably two typically schizophrenic symptoms (as specified for schizophrenia), diagnostic guidelines (a)–(d) should be clearly present.
This category should be used both for a single schizoaffective episode, depressive type, and for a recurrent disorder in which the majority of episodes are schizoaffective, depressive type.

F25.2 – Schizoaffective Disorder, Mixed Type

Symptoms of Schizophrenia (F20) co-exist with those of a mixed bipolar affective disorder (F31.6) should be coded.

F25.9 – Schizoaffective Disorder, Unspecified

No guidelines are listed.

F

Cheat Sheet: Schizophrenia

SCHIZOPHRENIA F20	F20.0 Paranoid Schizophrenia F20.2 Catatonic Schizophrenia F20.3 Undifferentiated Schizophrenia F20.9 Schizophrenia, Unspecified A fifth character may be used to classify the pattern of course: F20.x0 Continuous F20.x1 Episodic with progressive deficit F20x.9 Course uncertain, period of observation too short
Diagnostic Criteria and Guidelines • Thought distortions • Thought echo • Thought insertion • Thought broadcasting • Bizarre thoughts • Perception distortions • Delusions • Hallucinations • Disorganized speech	BLUE BOOK CRITERIA ONLY F20 - Schizophrenia The normal requirement for a diagnosis of schizophrenia is that a minimum of one very clear symptom (and usually two or more if less clear-cut) belonging to any one of the groups listed as (a) to (d) below, or symptoms from at least two of the groups referred to as (e) to (h), should have been clearly present for most of the time during a period of 1 month or more. Conditions meeting such symptomatic requirements but of duration less than 1 month (whether treated or not) should be diagnosed in the first instance as acute schizophrenia-like psychotic disorder and are classified as schizophrenia if the symptoms persist for longer periods.

- Strange use of words or way of speaking
- Catatonic behavior
- Social withdrawal
- Hostility or suspiciousness
- Anger
- Deterioration of personal hygiene
- Inappropriate
- Flat, expressionless gaze
- Inability to cry or express joy
- Inappropriate laughter or crying
- Oversleeping or insomnia
- Odd or irrational statements
- Forgetful; unable to concentrate
- Extreme reaction to criticism
- Depersonalization
- Derealization
- Somatic concerns
- Lack of insight/ awareness
- Impairments in motor coordination
- Impairments sensory integration
- Dishibitation
- Waxy
- Rigidity

a. thought echo, thought insertion or withdrawal, and thought broadcasting;
b. delusions of control, influence, or passivity, clearly referred to body or limb movements or specific thoughts, actions, or sensations; delusional perception;
c. hallucinatory voices giving a running commentary on the patient's behavior, or discussing the patient among themselves, or other types of hallucinatory voices coming from some part of the body;
d. persistent delusions of other kinds that are culturally inappropriate and completely impossible, such as religious or political identity, or superhuman powers and abilities (e.g. being able to control the weather, or being in communication with aliens from another world);
e. persistent hallucinations in any modality, when accompanied either by fleeting or half-formed delusions without clear affective content, or by persistent over-valued ideas, or when occurring every day for weeks or months on end;
f. breaks or interpolations in the train of thought, resulting in incoherence or irrelevant speech, or neologisms;
g. catatonic behavior, such as excitement, posturing, or waxy flexibility, negativism, mutism, and stupor;
h. "negative" symptoms such as marked apathy, paucity of speech, and blunting or incongruity of emotional responses, usually resulting in social withdrawal and lowering of social performance; it must be clear that these are not due to depression or to neuroleptic medication;
i. a significant and consistent change in the overall quality of some aspects of personal behavior, manifest as loss of interest, aimlessness, idleness, a self-absorbed attitude, and social withdrawal.
The diagnosis of schizophrenia should not be made in the presence of extensive depressive or manic symptoms unless it is clear that schizophrenic symptoms antedated the affective disturbance.

F20.1 Paranoid Schizophrenia

(a) delusions of persecution, reference, exalted birth, special mission, bodily change, or jealousy;
(b) hallucinatory voices that threaten the patient or give commands, or auditory hallucinations without verbal form, such as whistling, humming, or laughing;
(c) hallucinations of smell or taste, or of sexual or other bodily sensations; visual hallucinations may occur but are rarely predominant.
Thought disorder may be obvious in acute states, but if so it does not prevent the typical delusions or hallucinations from being described clearly. Affect is usually less blunted than in other varieties of schizophrenia, but a

minor degree of incongruity is common, as are mood disturbances such as irritability, sudden anger, fearfulness, and suspicion. "Negative" symptoms such as blunting of affect and impaired volition are often present but do not dominate the clinical picture.
The course of paranoid schizophrenia may be episodic, with partial or complete remissions, or chronic. In chronic cases, the florid symptoms persist over years and it is difficult to distinguish discrete episodes. The onset tends to be later than in the hebephrenic and catatonic forms.

F20.2 Catatonic Schizophrenia

The general criteria for a diagnosis of schizophrenia (see introduction to F20 above) must be satisfied. Transitory and isolated catatonic symptoms may occur in the context of any other subtype of schizophrenia, but for a diagnosis of catatonic schizophrenia one or more of the following behaviours should dominate the clinical picture:
1. stupor (marked decrease in reactivity to the environment and in spontaneous movements and activity) or mutism;
2. excitement (apparently purposeless motor activity, not influenced by external stimuli);
3. posturing (voluntary assumption and maintenance of inappropriate or bizarre postures);
4. negativism (an apparently motiveless resistance to all instructions or attempts to be moved, or movement in the opposite direction);
5. rigidity (maintenance of a rigid posture against efforts to be moved);
6. waxy flexibility (maintenance of limbs and body in externally imposed positions); and
7. other symptoms such as command automatism (automatic compliance with instructions), and perseveration of words and phrases.

F20.3 Undifferentiated Schizophrenia

Psychotic conditions meeting the general diagnostic criteria for schizophrenia but not conforming to any of the subtypes in F20.0–F20.2, or exhibiting the features of more than one of them without a clear predominance of a particular set of diagnostic characteristics.
(a) Meet the general criteria for schizophrenia;
(b) Either without sufficient symptoms to meet the criteria for only one of the subtypes F20.0, F20.1,F20.2, F20.4, or F20.5, or without so many symptoms that the criteria for more than one of the paranoid (F20.0), hebephrenic (F20.1)or catatonic (F20.2) subtypes are met.

F20.9 Schizophrenia, Unspecified (no guidelines listed).

G

Cheat Sheet: Schizophrenia Short Description

SCHIZOPHRENIA F20	F20.0 Paranoid Schizophrenia F20.2 Catatonic Schizophrenia F20.3 Undifferentiated Schizophrenia F20.9 Schizophrenia, Unspecified A fifth character may be used to classify the pattern of course: F20.x0 Continuous F20.x1 Episodic with progressive deficit F20x.9 Course uncertain, period of observation too short
Diagnostic Criteria and Guidelines • Thought distortions • Thought echo • Thought insertion • Thought broadcasting • Bizarre thoughts • Perception distortions • Delusions • Hallucinations • Disorganized speech • Strange use of words or way of speaking • Catatonic behavior • Social withdrawal	BLUE BOOK CRITERIA ONLY F20 - Schizophrenia The normal requirement for a diagnosis of schizophrenia is that a minimum of one very clear symptom (and usually two or more if less clear-cut) belonging to any one of the groups listed as (a) to (d) below, or symptoms from at least two of the groups referred to as (e) to (h), should have been clearly present for most of the time during a period of 1 month or more. Conditions meeting such symptomatic requirements but of duration less than 1 month (whether treated or not) should be diagnosed in the first instance as acute schizophrenia-like psychotic disorder and are classified as schizophrenia if the symptoms persist for longer periods.

- Hostility or suspiciousness
- Anger
- Deterioration of personal hygiene
- Inappropriate
- Flat, expressionless gaze
- Inability to cry or express joy
- Inappropriate laughter or crying
- Oversleeping or insomnia
- Odd or irrational statements
- Forgetful; unable to concentrate
- Extreme reaction to criticism
- Depersonalization
- Derealization
- Somatic concerns
- Lack of insight/ awareness
- Impairments in motor coordination
- Impairments sensory integration
- Dishibitation
- Waxy
- Rigidity

Index

For Product Safety Concerns and Information please contact our
EU representative GPSR@taylorandfrancis.com Taylor & Francis
Verlag GmbH, Kaufingerstraße 24, 80331 München, Germany